Thrive
The Bah! Guide to Wellness After cancer

STEPHANIE BUTLAND

Foreword by
David R. Hamilton PhD

HAY
HOUSE

HAY HOUSE
Australia • Canada • Hong Kong • India
South Africa • United Kingdom • United States

First published and distributed in the United Kingdom by:
Hay House UK Ltd, 292B Kensal Rd, London W10 5BE.
Tel.: (44) 20 8962 1230; Fax: (44) 20 8962 1239.
www.hayhouse.co.uk

Published and distributed in the United States of America by:
Hay House, Inc., PO Box 5100, Carlsbad, CA 92018-5100.
Tel.: (1) 760 431 7695 or (800) 654 5126; Fax: (1) 760 431 6948 or (800) 650 5115.
www.hayhouse.com

Published and distributed in Australia by:
Hay House Australia Ltd, 18/36 Ralph St, Alexandria NSW 2015.
Tel.: (61) 2 9669 4299; Fax: (61) 2 9669 4144.
www.hayhouse.com.au

Published and distributed in the Republic of South Africa by:
Hay House SA (Pty), Ltd, PO Box 990, Witkoppen 2068.
Tel./Fax: (27) 11 467 8904. www.hayhouse.co.za

Published and distributed in India by:
Hay House Publishers India, Muskaan Complex, Plot No.3, B-2,
Vasant Kunj, New Delhi – 110 070. Tel.: (91) 11 4176 1620; Fax: (91) 11 4176 1630.
www.hayhouse.co.in

Distributed in Canada by:
Raincoast, 9050 Shaughnessy St, Vancouver, BC V6P 6E5.
Tel.: (1) 604 323 7100; Fax: (1) 604 323 2600

Text © Stephanie Butland, 2012

The moral rights of the author have been asserted.

The information given in this book should not be treated as a substitute for professional medical advice; always consult a medical practitioner. Any use of information in this book is at the reader's discretion and risk. Neither the author nor the publisher can be held responsible for any loss, claim or damage arising out of the use, or misuse, or the suggestions made or the failure to take medical advice.

A catalogue record for this book is available from the British Library.

ISBN: 978-1-84850-966-5

Printed and bound in Great Britain by TJ International, Padstow, Cornwall.

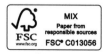

For Alan, Ned and Joy,
the lights of my life

Contents

Acknowledgements

When I was still calling myself a survivor, and wishing I could think of a better word for it, Natalie Jenkins told me she was 'thriving after cancer', and in doing so lightened my steps, made me smile and breathed life into the beginnings of this book.

A lot of people who are on the road to thriving took the time to answer my questions, and Anna, Natalie, Rachel, Keith, Liz, Gaynor, Jenny, Allison and Debbie agreed to be quoted. Thank you.

Dr David Hamilton understands exactly what this book is about. I'm so glad he wrote the foreword

Oli Munson of Blake Friedmann remains the Best Agent Ever. He even wears the hat I knitted him.

At Hay House, my editor Carolyn Thorne is intelligent, insightful and genuinely collaborative, and Jo Burgess and her team continue to be tirelessly enthusiastic on behalf of *Bah!*. Barbara Vesey did another fantastic job of copy-editing.

The work of Dr Edward de Bono first showed me that practical thinking strategies work, and matter.

My husband Alan, my children Ned and Joy and my parents Helen and Michael Breeze continue to be supporters, cheerleaders and sounding-boards in all that I do. I can't imagine thriving without them.

I owe sincere and special thanks to my friends for helping me to understand what I'm doing in these pages, and for doing it with such good grace, love, feedback, conversation, questions, coffee, cake and wine. Jude Evans, Nathalie Giauque, Kym Hadwin, Rebecca Leete, Scarlet Long, Emily Medland, Diane Mulholland, Louise Williams, I'm looking at you. Alan Butland and Susan Young, you are technically family, but the same goes for you.

Most importantly of all, *Bah!* blog and book readers remind me that I have something to say about cancer. I'm grateful to you and glad of your help. I hope the words in this book find you where you are, and help you to get to where you want to be.

Foreword

Thrive is a great word. It is so positive!

One of the things I love about Stephanie's writings is that they help you to feel empowered. It's all too easy to feel that we have no control over the circumstances of our lives, but Stephanie offers us a way to feel that there are things we can do, practical ways of acting, and healthy ways to think that give us a feeling that we can navigate our own course in life.

The mind is a powerful tool. I have written and spoken about it extensively. As a former scientist in the pharmaceutical industry, I became fascinated by the results of drugs trials where large numbers of ill people improved their health by taking placebos, even though the pills were often mostly sugar or blackboard chalk. It turns out that everything we think about alters the chemistry of our bodies.

So I love that Stephanie shares some visualizations in the book because they are a powerful way to use the mind. They are significant symbolic exercises, but in many ways the brain doesn't distinguish between real and imaginary. We know this from research at Harvard University where volunteers played a simple combination of piano notes for five consecutive days. Their brains were scanned every day and changes were noted as the brain responded to the movements – a phenomenon known as neuroplasticity. When the scans were placed side by side – those who played the notes and those who imagined them – they were almost identical. The brain had significantly changed in both cases. Imagination had actually changed brain structure. If we can do that, what else are we capable of doing?

That is such an empowering idea because it allows us to use our imaginations in any way we wish, and know that our imaginings are not empty, floaty things, but ideas that have real and potent effects in our bodies and our lives. The thought of thriving instead of surviving impacts how we think and alters the chemistry of our lives. It's about where we point the mind. Thriving seeds positive and creative ideas, strategies for navigating the often-difficult terrain of life, and it breeds hope and self-belief.

So I hope you enjoy reading this book. It is packed full of great ideas and numerous practical exercises, and it is written with a delightful and somewhat refreshing blend of good humour, common sense, honesty, and compassion that only a person who has gone through the experience of cancer and learned to thrive afterwards could write.

I hope you find what you need in this book and that it helps you to thrive.

David R. Hamilton PhD
Author of *How Your Mind Can Heal Your Body*

Introduction

*'You don't battle it, you endure it mostly –
a battle is quick and over with... this is a
long, drawn-out process.'*
Allison, diagnosed with breast cancer in 2009

I was diagnosed with a breast cancer in October 2008. I had the standard 'slash, poison and burn' treatment – surgery, chemotherapy and radiotherapy – and, if nothing continues to show on my annual mammograms and scans, the medical profession will announce me to be in remission five years from the date of surgery, on 18 November 2013. (I'm hoping for a party. I'll be disappointed if there aren't Nipples of Venus piled high on silver platters.)

The funny thing is that Official Remission Day will also be five years from the date that I came round from surgery and started to think of myself as cancer-free. There's the start of my occasionally tetchy relationship with the medical profession, right there. Medicine and I are like a health and safety consultant and a fire-eater thrashing out the details of a charity bungee-jump. We want the same outcome, but we're never going to agree on the details. (If you haven't already guessed, in that scenario I am the fire-eating would-be bungee-jumper. Which is fun for me on the page, because in Actual Real Life, bungee-jumping and fire-eating are pretty much at the top of the list of things you really couldn't pay me enough money to do. Along with being 17 again, living or working in any environment that involves being bitten by insects on a daily basis, and – um – having a cancer. Ah, yes. Back to the cancer.)

There are times during a dance with cancer when it feels as though everyone except you owns your body: every room you walk into seems to contain someone snapping on latex gloves in readiness for the next round of prodding, poking, needling and squeezing, accompanied by the questions you answered last week, and will answer again next week, about what your stomach, bowels, heart and lungs have been doing. With cancer the body is utterly subjugated, while dominating everything. It doesn't matter how well or terrible you feel, if the blood test results and the echocardiogram say you are well enough for treatment, you are well enough for treatment.

But my body wasn't the whole story of me, in the same way that yours isn't the total of you. To start with, I was shocked and surprised by how little interest cancer treatment and cancer professionals had in what went on in the heads of patients. (Maybe they just assumed it was something along the lines of 'Please don't let me die, and is that needle absolutely necessary?' – which, to be fair, wouldn't be too far from the truth, most of the time.) But fortunately for my sanity, I cottoned on fairly fast to the fact that, by and large, nobody cared what was happening in my head, provided that it wasn't a metastasizing lump of cancer. Nobody owned my mind but *me*. And because I work with the mind, I knew just how much what went on in my head mattered.

And so I thought my way through cancer, and I blogged my way through it, too. I wrote a book, *How I Said Bah! To cancer: a guide to living, laughing, thinking and dancing your way through*, and lots of magazines and charities and book reviewers said lovely things about it, but what really mattered to me was what other people who had danced with cancer had to say. 'As someone with terminal cancer I found this book very lifting... what a refreshing read... Many ideas within the book I've adopted and as a result feel a lot more contented with the situation I'm finding myself in,' wrote one Amazon reviewer. Another said, 'I was struggling but feel this author [is] so spot on she could have been following me around. Great lift.' On the blog someone commented, 'I want to thank you. You have allowed me to tweak those final wee pieces of my mind which were bugging me... This is a great book, funny [and] real.' GPs contacted me to say they were recommending it to their patients; patients told me that they'd bought copies for their oncologists. I am proud of what the *Bah!* book is doing in the world. But I finished writing it a little under two years after diagnosis, and something very important has happened since then: I've stopped thinking my way through treatment, and found that now I need to think my way through wellness. Which is as much of a challenge, at times. But if this book has found its way into your hand, you probably already know that.

Welcome to *Thrive: the Bah! guide to wellness after cancer*.

******

Statistics vary, but it's reasonable to assume that, somewhere in the world, one person dies every one minute from a cancer. Every minute, another family closes its eyes because, in that instant of loss, looking at the world is too much. Every minute, the long journey through shock and anger and disbelief and depression and being unable to remember and incapable of forgetting and bargaining with the universe and struggling through every wretched and bloody day begins for another group of people who have lost someone that they love.

Of course, not all cancers, not all people with a cancer, not all families, not all deaths are alike. I hear a lot of stories about how people cope with the dying days of cancer. Relatives and friends talk through last minutes, days, hours, in frame-by-frame forensic detail, knowing that this story is one to be told well, told properly, not hurried through or snatched at. Nothing can be skimmed over. Everything matters: the drugs, the setting, the colour of the skin, the opening and closing of the eyes, the food rejected, the sleep and the little bouts of laughter, the ability of the fingers to touch, to hold, to let go.

Some people thrash and cling to stay with their families. Someone I know took his wife's hand and told her that it was all right for her life to end now. That he and their children would manage without her somehow, though it wasn't, oh it wasn't, what they wanted. That it was time for her to be free of the pain she was in. She needed that permission to close her eyes and die, and she did, right at that moment. Some people refuse medical intervention and let nature take its course, hoping that, on balance, the quality of their remaining days will outweigh the quantity, if they opt out of the harsh and unrelenting treatments that are the only, tiny, hope of saving them. (I don't think that the phrase 'kill or cure' was invented for late-stage chemotherapy treatments, but it's certainly a cap that fits.)

Others are wheeled into the chemotherapy unit even though they are so ill that a nurse must support their head to help them to take an anti-sickness drug before another round of treatment, the one that they hope will contain that tiny drop of miracle, begins. Some people, given months to live by a doctor, die on the day that has been predicted for them, as though it was a target or an inevitability. For some, the end is sudden, a matter of days between the diagnosis from the ever-encroaching cluster of symptoms and swellings; for others, death comes at the end of years and years of having cancer close at hand. I've known people who disappear from life before they have truly gone, choosing final weeks of near-solitude and hoping that the people whose lives they have been part of will remember them as the someone before their skin became the colour of putty and it hurt to open their eyes. And I've known – we've all known – the ones who put on their lipstick, learn to ride a wheelchair and go out into the world to tell it to make cancer stop.

But alongside this host of the dead and dying, there's an ever-increasing crowd of people like me. The survivors. The ones who were lucky enough to find an obvious symptom early, and sensible enough to tell someone about it, and that someone in their turn was sensible enough to send them to the doctor to be on the safe side. The ones who had a bottom-of-the-class cancer that hadn't yet figured out that the lymphatic system is a high-speed rail-link around the body to lots of other places that would be happy to host a cancer, too. The ones who submitted themselves to a cure which was worse than the disease.

One of the funny-peculiar things about cancer – and, of course, what makes it so very dangerous – is the lack of symptoms in the early stages. So people like me feel perfectly well when they, in fact, have a swiftly growing lump getting ready to make a major assault on them. And then the process of curing us from this painless, innocuous thing makes us, very possibly, more ill than we have ever been in our lives. 'Be brave!' say the people who've never had chemotherapy. 'It's not as bad as chemotherapy!' say the people who've never had radiotherapy. 'Yes', we say, and we submit, feeling as though this is all the wrong way round, surely, like eating dessert first? Except that eating dessert first feels good, at least until you try to get into last summer's shorts.

There was a time, not so very long ago, when a cancer diagnosis meant that, if you were lucky, you probably had just about enough time to dig out your will and iron your pyjamas before you began The Final Journey. Fortunately, it isn't like that anymore, Better education, better diagnostics, better treatments mean that more and more people are surviving cancer. And surviving it for a looooong time. Some of us are lucky enough to get away with the annual screening. (And of course the borderline-obsessive feeling for lumps in the interim. I doubt that I'm the only breast cancer survivor who's been told off by their daughter for doing some unconscious breast-poking, complete with analytical gazing-into-middle-distance face, in public.) Others have regular recurrences that are fairly easily contained – necks of bladders and cervixes seem especially good breeding-grounds for small clumps of stay-at-home cancers. Yet others have more drastic recurrences and spend their lives going round the cancer conveyer belt over and over again. The fact is, more of us are surviving cancer than dying from it. Which means that there are plenty of us who are wandering around with a nagging feeling that we shouldn't really be here. Culturally there's still a part of us that thinks surviving cancer is a bit of freakish good fortune – the medical equivalent of having a cannonball go right through your middle, cartoon-style, and living to tell the tale – so, often, it's hard to know how to 'do' life after cancer.

So, what happens? Well, we get re-assimilated into our worlds when treatment stops. We get back our hair, or sometimes new hair, more abundant or more curly or more brittle or more grey. We go back to work, and after a few weeks everyone stops telling us how well we look, and they say, 'How are you?' as an everyday 'don't-really-tell-me-because-I'm-just-being-polite-and-I'm-actually-rather-busy' way, rather than 'How ARE you?' with head on one side and full eye contact and one hand touching you lightly just above the elbow. We slot back into our old roles and our old relationships, except maybe at Christmas parties and impromptu Friday night trips to the pub, when someone sits down next to us and tells us how shocked they were and how brave we are and how glad they are that we're alive. (And, if it's late, how much they really, really love us.) Those little cancer privileges we get at home – ironing exemptions, tea on demand (or before-demand), queen of the TV remote control – gradually slip away. So do the moments when you look up from a book and find a member of your family looking at you as though you are a minor deity/they are a Dickensian orphan.

As cancer fades into memory, we can complain of a headache without someone calling the out-of-hours emergency oncologist on speed dial. The out-of-hours emergency oncologist's number isn't transferred when we get a new phone. We can phone someone without them sounding a little bit panicky when they hear who's on the end of the line. We have our haircut and no one comments, because haircuts have become ordinary again. (To the outsider, at least. A year and a half on from my first post-chemotherapy haircut and I still can't sleep the night before a trim, from sheer excitement. Honestly. It sounds ridiculous – maybe it is ridiculous – but it's true.)

So, we have Survived. Things are Back To Normal. We can all Breathe A Sigh Of Relief and Thank Our Lucky Stars and Say All The Other Things That We Say As A Way Of Saying Something When We Don't Know Quite What To Say.

Except.

BLOG POST, 16 JANUARY 2011: THE WAY TO SAY IT

You will know, if you read Bah! regularly, that although I am pleased and proud to be a breast cancer survivor, I don't really like the word survivor. There's a certain joylessness to it, I find. (After all, someone who crawls from the wreckage of a car crash with multiple fractures and missing an eye has survived the accident.)

Natalie already helped me out a great deal this week when she told me she was a 16-year breast cancer survivor. But then she put something in the comments that helped me even more:

'Next time I'll say… "I've been thriving for over 16 years since my breast cancer diagnosis!" Which is a more accurate description of my journey.'

Thrive. That's the word I've been searching for.

Although I knew what it meant, I was so enamoured of it that I looked it up in a dictionary:

thrive |θrīv| verb

(of a child, animal, or plant) grow or develop well or vigorously: the new baby thrived • prosper; flourish: education groups thrive on organization [as adj.] (thriving) a thriving economy.

ORIGIN Middle English (originally in the sense [grow, increase]): from Old Norse thrífask, reflexive of thrífa 'grasp, get hold of.'

You gotta love those origins. A cross between 'grow' and 'get hold of' feels like exactly what I've been doing for the last two and a bit years. (And eating biscuits. And knitting.)

A bit giddy, I went to the thesaurus next:

thrive

flourish, prosper, burgeon, bloom, blossom, mushroom, do well, advance, succeed, boom.

What a fabulous parade of words that is.

I'm not going to tell people I'm a breast cancer survivor any more. I'm going to say, 'I was diagnosed with a breast cancer in 2008, I had treatment, and now I'm thriving.' For variety, I might say 'flourishing' from time to time. (I'll stay away from mushrooming, advancing and booming, I think.)

Of course, there have been weeks and months when I've felt like that unfortunate person dragging themselves from the wreck of a car: there have been times when I have been a breast cancer survivor, at best, and if you'd asked me whether I felt I was thriving I'd have held up a piece of paper saying 'hollow laughter' because I wouldn't have had the energy to actually laugh. There may be times to come when I feel like a survivor again. But right now, I'm thriving. I wish you thriving too.

******

We might feel that we must have, now, a life of brilliant days and the kind of nights that F. Scott Fitzgerald would write about if he was in a really, really good mood: all cocktails, bubbling laughter and azure skies. We might feel the burden of having lived when others have died and, if we chose to, we could wonder, every minute, why we are alive and why we aren't ecstatic.

The trouble – or rather, the fact – is that cancer is a traumatic experience even when we do survive it. It is, in the truest sense, life-changing. Look at me. As direct or indirect results of dancing with cancer, I've changed my career, I've moved to the other end of the country and I've lost the really annoying kink in my fringe. I've kept my family and most of my friends, and I've relaxed. A lot. In the TV show of 'Stephanie's Top 50 Most Life-Changing Moments Ever', viewed only by insomniacs, people with brand new babies and those who have lost the remote control, cancer is going to be way up at the top, after the final commercial break.

And you don't change your life without there being emotional fall-out. In other words, after cancer it's OK to wake up in the morning and not want to pick flowers, embrace strangers and throw an impromptu tea party that people will talk about for months because it was just so sparklingly, effortlessly brilliant. It's OK – it's even normal – to feel odd and disconnected and unsure. It's fine to feel a little bit estranged from the person you were before you found the lump or had the headache or went to the doctor because you just felt so grim. Because you are different now. There are millions of us around the world making a post-cancer life.

This book is meant to help you to get from survival to a place where you are thriving. I hope it will help you in finding your new, post-cancer self, and figure out a comfortable space in the world. In these pages you'll find thinking techniques and strategies, visualizations, meditations, questions, candour and common sense. Please, as you read this book, take what is for you and leave what is not. What I recommend is that you read it once, quickly, from start to finish, then find or buy yourself a beautiful 'Thriving Notebook' and go back and work your way through the parts that you need, as you need them.

Journey well, and be well, and continue to be well.

BAH! THINKING

A visualization for life after cancer

Become comfortable: sit or lie down, relax and close your eyes.

Breathe. Breathe in through your nose and out through your mouth. Start with five big inhalations and exhalations, and then let your breath come and go at a slow and steady pace. Breathing might feel like the water lapping on a beach, or a pendulum swinging back and forth. Just breathe.

When you are ready, turn your thoughts to cancer. Visualize it. Visualize it in a way that feels true to all of the difficulty it has given you. Maybe it's an ogre, or a sinister clown. Perhaps it takes the form of a ghoul or a shadow or an angry-looking cloud, a grabbing, pinching goblin, a wailing waif. Allow yourself to see it, to face it, even to be afraid of it. Keep breathing that comfortable, rhythmical breath.

Now imagine yourself turning your back on this monstrous cancer. Imagine yourself walking away. Be aware that the cancer isn't following you. Realize that it cannot follow you. It's stuck in the time and place where it accosted you. But you are free. You can move. You have the power in your limbs, the power in your heart, the will to leave this thing behind you. Do it. Breathe. Breathe. Keep breathing. Walk away from the cancer. Keep walking. Feel the distance between you and cancer grow, and expand, and be filled with light.

Smile. Breathe.

Feel how good that distance feels.

When you are ready, open your eyes.

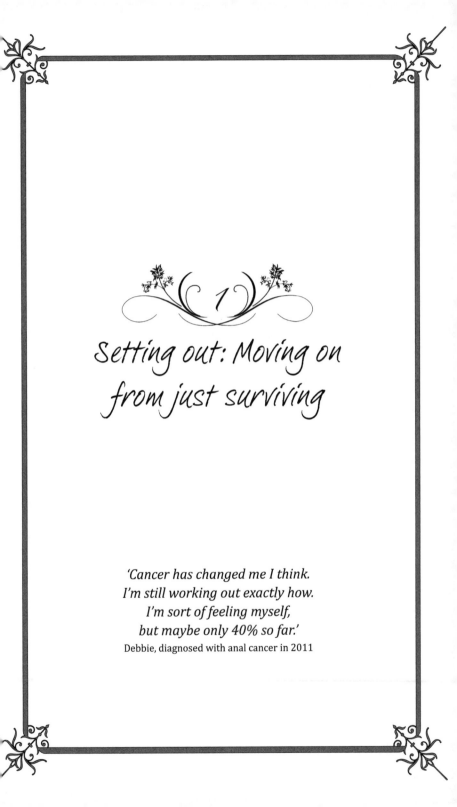

1

Setting out: Moving on from just surviving

'Cancer has changed me I think.
I'm still working out exactly how.
I'm sort of feeling myself,
but maybe only 40% so far.'
Debbie, diagnosed with anal cancer in 2011

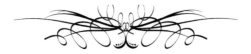

I don't think that anyone really thinks they're going to die. Or, more accurately: no one really thinks they're going to die today. Or tomorrow. Sometime, yes of course, absolutely. But that 'sometime' is a long way off. Because we all have things to do. People to love. Places to go. Books to write, songs to sing, kisses to kiss, socks to knit. (OK, that last one's probably more specific to me than the others are.)

A dance with cancer means a whole swathe of time during which you get to think about dying. Even if the diagnosis is relatively good – yes, the cancer is there, but it looks small and manageable – death watches from the sidelines as we dance with cancer, whether we want him to or not. Because even with a straightforward diagnosis, no medic will ever say, 'You're not going to die.' They go for something like, 'The prognosis is excellent.' They can't actually tell you that you're not going to die, because you always might, for example, get hit by one of those buses of 'you might get hit by a bus tomorrow' fame. You might pick up something nasty while you're on the ward. You might have more cancer than there first appears. So they tell you 'the prognosis is excellent' as shorthand for 'all else being equal – which of course it isn't – and 'assuming that what we have seen is all there is to see (which we can't assume at all), there's a good chance you'll live to tell this tale.' That's as much of a guarantee as you're going to get and, if I were you, I'd take it. But it's all about 'not dying'. And the trouble is, words to the effect of 'you're unlikely to die' have the same effect on your brain as 'you're unlikely to have salmon for dinner.' What happens when your boeuf bourgignon arrives? That's right: all you can think about is salmon.

So it is with cancer and death. For those of us surviving, every day of treatment is less about being alive and more about being not-dead. And the fact that there are days when treatment makes you feel half-dead doesn't help you to think about the big D any less, whether consciously or unconsciously. I was once on an oncology ward having day treatment when one of the people in the side wards died. The porters came to collect the body and, as it was wheeled out, there wasn't really any sense of shock from those of us that remained. Sorrow, yes, and regret, but also a sense that, well, this was what cancer could, and would, and frequently did, do. The nurses closed the doors on to the side rooms and the body was wheeled through an empty, silent corridor. Everyone stopped what they were doing as it passed. Some of us closed our eyes.

When the nurses re-opened the doors, that was our cue to look each other in the eyes and exchange looks that were a mixture of sadness, understanding and a sense of 'there but for the grace of God go I'. Then there was a general sigh, and we all went back to what we'd been doing: not dying.

I think one of the first signs of survival – in the properly, vibrantly alive sense, rather than the 'yup, according to the condensation on the surface of this mirror, I am still breathing' sense – is that you finally stop thinking of yourself as being Not Dead all the time. Being alive ceases to be the daily miracle and becomes again the daily bread. And that's the point at which you are ready to think about what happens next.

******

Somewhere towards the end of 2010 I decided to start talking about wellness: to take a positive step with the language I was using, in my head to myself as well as out loud to others, and to abandon the idea that not being ill, not being dead, was good enough.

This shift came partly, I think, because I was ready for it, and partly because I reached the stage in recovery where hardly a day passed without me thinking about how I was doing something I couldn't do at that time the previous year.

They weren't spectacular things. One day I lugged a three-days' suitcase through a busy railway station, keeping up with the sweep of travellers, not having to get myself to the edges of the human traffic to take a breather. Increasingly I would take a walk just for the sake of taking a walk, and without panicking that I'd gone too far to be able to get back without being a tearful wreck. (Generally, I noticed, two years on from diagnosis I was spending a lot less time in a state of tearful wreckage.) The meals I decided to cook, the cakes I baked, weren't decided according to how long I thought I could spend on my feet in one go. Sometimes I'd follow a day at work with a drink with colleagues instead of a bone-weary trudge of a journey home and an evening of struggling to keep my eyes open. Cancer stopped being a necessary part of conversation – explaining why I was bald/sitting down/drinking milk/had a load of medical kit hanging out of my arm – and became something I mentioned if I wanted to. In fairness to myself, I should say that there was one spectacular thing, in September 2009, and then again in September 2010. I walked 20 miles through London at night to raise money for Maggie's Cancer Caring Centres. The first time it took nearly 12 hours and it took me two weeks to recover. I still have a scar on the bottom of my foot from the 5-inch blister. The second time, my son, my dad and I took 9 hours to do it. I've seldom been so proud – of myself, of the people who walked with me, the ones I knew and the ones that I didn't.

All of these things meant that I felt well. And so I changed my response to the question, 'How are you?' I stopped saying, 'Not bad', or 'I'm doing OK.' Instead I said, 'I'm very, very well.' Granted, my definition was only just going to scrape through as a way of talking about wellness – I can breathe! I can walk! I can stay up until 10 p.m. most nights! I don't feel 'looked after' everywhere I go! – but it felt like wellness to me.

BAH! THINKING

A record of wellness

Take yourself, a notebook and a pen to a quiet place where you won't be disturbed.

Ignore the first page of the notebook and turn to the first double-page spread.

At the top of the left-hand side of the page, write the date and then, 'Wellness is...', and make a list of everything that, right now, means that you are well, to you. It doesn't matter whether wellness is being able to put on your own shoes without help, or leaving the house more than once a day, or running a marathon.

Read that list back. Read it out loud. Feel proud.

Now, at the top of the right-hand side of the page, write 'Wellness will be...' and make another list, of the things that are just out of your reach: the things that will mean real progress when you can do them.

Read that list back. Read it out loud. Feel excited about what's possible.

Revisit this list regularly: say, once a month. Put a date in your diary, take out your notebook and read through what wellness was a month ago and what you were aiming for. Turn the page and repeat the exercise. There's a good chance that a lot of what was on the right-hand page last month has made its way onto the left-hand page this time. If it has, great. If it hasn't, it might go onto the right-hand page again. Or it might not matter anymore. This list isn't here to make you feel inadequate, or in competition with yourself: it's here to show your progress, to yourself, so that on days when you feel as though you'll never be really well again... you'll be able to prove to yourself that you already are.

I'm a great believer in having A Plan. Even if the plan changes on an almost hourly basis, I still like to have one. Although in one light my dance with cancer has shown me how little control I really have over my life – it sure as hell screwed my diary for the back end of 2008 and most of 2009 – in another, it has shown me how important having a plan is.

A plan shows you where you're going. A plan gives you purpose. A plan gives you something to aim for. Almost everyone I know who is successful is someone who plans. Just in case that last sentence makes you think you've picked up the wrong book, please let me clarify. By 'successful' I don't mean one of those fierce types you see on TV who sold their first company at the age of 20 for £20 million, has teeth so white you can perform surgery on a kitten by their light alone, and says things like 'Sleep is for the weak.' By 'successful' I mean whatever feels like achievement to you. It might be how you feel, what you earn, what you do, who you spend your time with.

For months, success for me was simply the fact that I was Not Dead and Not Dying.

But there comes a point when that changes. That's the beginning of the journey to thriving.

BAH! THINKING

A visualization for working out what you want

Find somewhere quiet, get comfortable and breathe deeply. When you are ready, close your eyes.

In your mind, see yourself walking along a path through a forest. You can hear the wind ruffling the branches above you; the air is warm; your feet make the next step effortlessly.

In your mind, walk this path until you're in a state of tranquillity.

Imagine turning a corner to see a hut in front of you. Push open the door and go in.

Find yourself in a room lined with shelves, and the shelves filled with everything you could ever want: objects that you might want for themselves, but also objects that symbolize places, adventures, people.

Keep breathing deeply. In your mind, see yourself turn slowly in this room stuffed with possibility. In your mind, allow yourself to reach out and start to take things from the shelves, putting the objects you choose at your feet. Allow yourself not to know what you're going to choose until it's in your hand.

When you have enough, take up your choices, turn around, leave the hut and let the door close behind you.

Open your eyes.

Write down what you've chosen.

The first time I did what you've just done – after having done something similar at a conference sometime before – I found that I had a book, written by me, in my hand.

BAH! THINKING
A plan for thriving

It's time to turn to that list of wishes and possibilities, and make it into a plan.

First, take the list, and take another look. Look at everything on the list and see if there's anything there that isn't realistic, or serious. Buying winning lottery tickets, bringing people back from the dead, being 6 inches taller, that sort of thing. Take them off the list. (These thinking strategies are good, but they're not that good.)

Now take a moment to think about every item that remains on the page, in turn. Think about whether it's really something you want to do, or whether it's something you think you want, or ought to want. If you really want it, it stays. If not, it goes. Life is short, whether it is shortened by cancer or not. Let's not spend time striving to get to somewhere only to find we'd rather be at home.

When you have your final list, sit back and take a look at it. Consider what's there, and put an asterisk next to the three things that are most important to you. These are the things that you're going to work on.

For each of the three things, do the following:

Take a fresh page. Write at the top: 'I will achieve x by date.'

Underneath, write down the ten steps you will take in order to get you to that goal.

Remember, this is not a race, or a competition. You could write 'I will complete my novel within ten years' and have a smaller step towards that of 'I will write ten words a day.' Or you could have 'I will become a qualified carpenter/aromatherapist/lion-tamer by the end of the decade,' with steps that break down into saving the money, doing the research and taking the course part-time over five years. What we are trying to do here is to create achievable goals that will get you, little by little, towards what you really want.

Review your steps often. Add new ones, break them down further, skip steps that are no longer necessary. This tool is your slave, not your master. The important thing is that you are doing something towards your goal every day.

Let's take a joke break.

A man wants to win the lottery. Every day he walks up a hill to the church near his home, and he prays for an hour: 'Please, Lord, let me win the lottery.' After a year, he increases his prayer time to two hours; after another year, to three: 'Please, Lord, let me win the lottery.' Eventually, he is on his knees for five hours a day: 'Please, Lord, let me win the lottery.' One day the man is at prayer as usual when suddenly the skies darken, there's a crack of lightning and God himself appears before the cowering supplicant. And God says: 'Help me out here. Why don't you GO AND BUY A TICKET?'

In other words – you have to help yourself.

BLOG POST, 14 JANUARY 2009: 5 YEARS FROM NOW

Last night over dinner, Alan asked me where I'd like to be in 5 years' time. (I don't think it was a job interview. If it was, my lengthy discourses on the merits of knitting hats and the frustrations of daytime TV scheduling may have scuppered my chances.)

I said (in no particular order):

1. I would like to be well, and for our family to be well.

2. I would like to be with you. (This was not only a politically expedient answer, but also true.)

3. I would like to have seen the Northern Lights. (If there was an order [to this list], this would be at the top. I've wanted to see the Northern Lights for as long as I can remember.)

4. I would like to be known as an authority on de Bono's work, and to be spending my working time on de Bono.

5. I would like to have published at least one book.

6. I would like to own one of Anita Klein's angels...

That was it. I suspect that if I'd been asked that question four months ago, the list would have been much longer, much less focused, and probably quite a lot less realistic. Dancing with cancer has made me realize that while my previous scattergun approach to life (training! networking! cakes! psychology degree! scuba diving! very long list of holiday destinations!) may have been fun, it might not be satisfying. (A bit like how, in the long term, a mushroom risotto makes a better dinner than a packet of Kettle Chips and a double chocolate muffin.)

I'll keep you posted as I knock things off the list.

******

Here's how I'm doing with the list, three years on at time of writing. 1 is going well, 2 is too, and is still true, 3 still needs to happen, 4 has shifted a little, because of 5 happening. And I've done 6. There's a beautiful blue angel, releasing a bird, hanging over our fireplace in the living room. It makes me smile every time I look at it. And when I turned 40, my friends gave me another angel, smiling against a starry sky.

******

So, now you have a plan.

I've got a plan too, and you're welcome to adapt it as part of your own.

Here it is:

Let's have no more talk of death.

Out of the woods:
When treatment is
(almost) over

*'I define wellness as not being prevented by
my body from doing anything I want to do.'*
Rachel, diagnosed with breast cancer in 2008

BLOG POST, 22 APRIL 2010:
THAT'S NOT MY NAME

I think language is important. I believe that the words that we choose reach out into the world and show the world how to treat us. And I believe that those words also snake down into our unconscious and form a blueprint for our brains to follow. As Henry Ford said, 'Whether you think you can or whether you think you can't, you are right.'

Right from the beginning of my dance with cancer, I've chosen my words with care. I've never had cancer, I've had a cancer. It's always been the cancer, it's never been my cancer. It's been a dance, not a fight.

I've struggled to find a way to talk about myself, though, through this dance. 'Victim', obviously, is a non-starter, as is 'fighter' (though I can see why it works for other people). Out there in the world are people who call themselves cancer vixens or breast cancer babes, which I admire, but am not convinced I could pull off. I've ended up defaulting to 'survivor' but it's not really satisfactory. There's something a bit 'thank goodness we managed to lash a raft together out of the corpses of our friends' about it. And not a lot of joie de vivre.

So, trying to find a way to describe myself used to be tricky. But lately – especially over the last few weeks, as Herceptin side-effects fade and strength begins to return – it's got easier.

Who am I? I'm Stephanie. It's as simple as that.

Well, almost. I'm not quite the same Stephanie who walked into St George's Hospital to have surgery just over 18 months ago. But a lot of me is the same. Some of me is worse, and some of me is better. As Ernest Hemingway said, 'The world breaks everyone, and afterward, some are strong at the broken places.' I think I'm mostly stronger.

And now I'm a Stephanie who finds that she can be just herself again. Now the answer to questions like, 'What have you been up to' or 'How are you feeling' or 'What are your plans for the summer' do not need to have a reference to cancer in the answer. I'm quite happy to 'fess up to breast cancer': so much of what I do now is borne out of that dance. But I think it's time to leave the labels behind.

******

There comes a time when treatment is, if not over, then feeling a bit over. The needles are decreasing in both size and frequency, the hair is returning, appointments dwindle from twice-weekly to weekly to monthly to six-monthly. People start saying things like 'back to normal' and 'glad it's over'. And it's lovely. In a way. And they're right. To a degree.

But.

It's not over.

Treatment for cancer re-calibrates your idea of what's an acceptable level of medical intervention, so it's possible to find yourself in a situation where you, the person dancing-with-cancer-but-now-generally-deemed-to-be-well-again-by-everyone, are still having treatment that only looks like nothing because you've had so much worse done to you in the name of a cure.

This, for me, was one of the hardest things about my dance with cancer. There were points when treatment became less invasive, and I felt everyone around me relax and get back to their lives. Which was, to an extent, something that I was glad about. But there was a part of me – the part that was swallowing daily tablets that were inducing a five-year medical menopause, for example – that struggled to see everyone else behaving as though something that was a big deal for me, didn't much matter to them.

Of course, it wasn't that it didn't much matter. It was that I was downplaying the side-effects and how I felt about them. I was as guilty of re-calibrating what I thought was worth making a fuss about as everyone else. I did, eventually, figure out that inwardly seething was not the way to address this. (I'm not always as quick on the uptake as I could be.)

The thing that really helped me to see this was writing a blog post about how lousy I was feeling. I don't often do that. I do blog posts about how today isn't great, but tomorrow will be better, or blog posts about what a good plan it is to have a breast cancer at a time in history when medicine, albeit unpleasant medicine, can get you back to your life. I do blog posts about how I feel lousy and then I do something about it. So writing a thoroughly sorry-for-myself miserable blog post was unusual, and as I hit the 'publish' button I felt more anxious and vulnerable than I do on the days when I post a poem or a photograph of my breasts.

Within hours of the post going up, these things had happened:

- I'd had dozens of emails and comments offering me encouragement and support, including one message asking for my address so the sender could send me some yarn, which they did.

- My Beloved Auntie Susan (to give her her full title) texted me to remind me to 'Remember, one more step along the way I go…'

- Alan left work, came home and kept me company.

- My friend Nathalie rang to check on me, and then came over to give me a hug.

- Joy and I cuddled up on the sofa, ate chocolate and chatted.

- I was forgiven my earlier grumpiness, which had been spectacular, possibly even award-winning.

All of which meant that I learned that I don't have to suffer on my own, and that it's normal – OK, even – to be brought down by antibiotics, anxiety and aching. But I only got the help that I needed by taking the first step – admitting that I felt terrible. It was hard. It gets easier.

BAH! THINKING

Strategies for keeping connected

- *Schedule a weekly meeting, or a time to talk about how you are feeling about your treatment.*

- *Resist the temptation to trill 'I'm fine! Absolutely fine! Never better!' when people ask you how treatment is going and how you are feeling. People will want to believe you, because they want you to be well. Don't expect them to suss out the subtext and/or notice and question the note of slight hysteria in your voice. Cancer doesn't absolve you from responsibility for yourself.*

- *Learn when things are likely to be difficult for you and forewarn/remind people when those times are coming up. In my family, everyone knew when Herceptin Day came around and did their best to look after me then, but actually it was the day before when I needed support. On those days I was dreading treatment and really wishing I didn't have to have it because I'd been playing at being well for a fortnight since the last side-effects subsided; on those days I needed looking after. Something that I routinely forgot about until it was too late, everyone was at work/school, and I was having a little cry on my own and not wanting to upset anyone by ringing them and wailing at them. And promising myself I would remember next time. Which I generally didn't.*

- *Have a noticeboard or place in your house where you can show how you are all feeling today. A blackboard where you can draw a smiling, or unsmiling, face, a flower, a sunshine, a storm cloud, would work. And/or have a place where anyone in the household can write down what they need help with. Sometimes it's easier to write it than say it.*

- *Remember that you're not the only person with challenges and difficulties in their lives. Cancer is rubbish, yes, and the seemingly endless bits of treatment and then recovery are boring and awful and you need a bit of looking after, of course you do. But if you're 13 and you've fallen out with your best friend, or you're 15 and you have an exam tomorrow, or if you're any age you care to pick and it's the anniversary of your father's death or you have a toothache, well, no matter how much that person loves you and cares for you, you aren't going to be at the forefront of their heart. Accept this, rejoice in the wider world you're part of, and save your worries and stresses for later. The chances are that a lot of people have done the same for you since your dance with cancer began.*

- *If you're struggling, do something about it straight away. I've lost count of the times I've kept going, only to eventually have a big wobble and a cry, and then immediately be greeted with a concerned: 'Why didn't you say something sooner?'*

- *Have a code word that will ensure that you are taken seriously when you need to be. I found that 'I'm feeling a bit low' would sometimes get me a 'there, there' reaction when I needed something more. Something I've suggested that others try is establishing a code word that means 'I really need you to put down whatever it is that you're doing, no matter how important, and help me right now.' Someone I've worked with says, 'I'm feeling tomato' when she needs her husband to notice that she's struggling. (Neither of them like tomatoes. Feel free to choose the mutually repellant fruit, vegetable, or other item of your choice.)*

As I was writing this chapter I started to wonder exactly why it is that I find asking for help so hard. So I sat down and made a list of the possibilities:

23

1. I'm afraid that if I'm too much of a bother to people, they'll stop loving me.

2. I don't want to turn into one of those characters from a period drama – nothing wrong with them except their belief that if they move more than three feet from their chaise longue they'll have some sort of nervous collapse. And I believe that the best way to avoid this is to pretend I'm OK when I'm not.

3. I don't want to be ill. So I'm averse to doing anything that suggests I'm ill. Asking for help is one of those things, as it means I'm admitting to not feeling 100%.

I suspect that, actually, my aversion to asking for help is a combination of these three elements, each of which is quite a challenge in its own right. Although I haven't 'solved' any of my list, being aware of it does make me feel a bit more forgiving of myself. If you find asking for help difficult, too, it might be a good idea to think about why. (If you find asking for help easy, maybe you should be writing a book about how you do it. I'll be right at the front of the queue to buy it.)

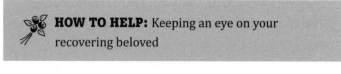

HOW TO HELP: Keeping an eye on your recovering beloved

- Know the signs. You'll know your loved one well enough to know that silence, or incessant talking, or getting up at 4:30 a.m., or a sudden interest in really terrible TV is a sign that they are having a difficult time. As soon as you think something might be wrong, ask.

- Don't be afraid to challenge. Most of us are programmed to answer the question, 'Are you all right?' with 'Yes', the first time. Check. Ask again. Say, 'You don't seem all right to me.' (Say it in a nice way.)

- Pre-empt. Look out for those days or times or bits of treatment that might make your beloved tetchy or unwell or sad. Don't leave them alone; arrange nice but non-taxing treats; provide a distraction – a new book, renting a DVD they missed at the cinema. (If you can do this without making it seem like a big deal, so much the better.)

- Involve them in your life. Don't hide your problems or pretend you've just had a perfect day if you haven't. Share your frustrations. Your relationship will outlive cancer, and in order for it to do that in a healthy way, you need to take as well as give.

- Start conversations about cancer… because cancer is part of your shared history now, whatever your relationship is. It's all right to talk about it; and it's useful for the person who is recovering from it to feel that they are not the only one who's been profoundly affected. But these don't need to be deep and meaningful conversations: recall funny things, incidental things. It's a bit like coping with bereavement, I think: it's healthier to talk about the person you have lost than to pretend that they never existed, although, in the short term, the pretence would probably be easier.

My mum and I still laugh about the nurse who delayed the removal of my post-surgery dressings so that she could tell us, with all the seriousness of a 5-year-old explaining exactly how letters get to Father Christmas, about the sandwich she had just had, which wasn't very nice. (I will spare you the details. I wasn't really paying a lot of attention, to be honest, because I was trying to work out how it was that I had come to be sitting in a windowless room, naked from the waist up and bruised to all hell, listening to someone I'd never met talk about their lunch.)

BAH! THINKING

Taking responsibility

Take that trusty notebook and find a fresh double-page spread.

Write 'I can control' at the top of the left-hand page.

Make a list of all the things that are both important to you and completely within your control. The list might include what you eat, what you read, when you sleep, what you listen to, where you go, how and when you exercise, who you spend time with... or none of those things might matter in your world. Create your list.

On the right-hand page, write 'I choose...', and for each item on the left, write down something that will help you. For example, if 'I can control when I sleep' is on the left, the entries on the right might be 'I will go to bed as soon as I feel tired' or 'I will get up at 7 a.m. every day' or 'I will take a sleeping tablet if I don't get to sleep within half an hour of going to bed.' Or all three. This is about creating ways to help you to make the best possible world to start thriving in.

Now find another double-page spread. On the left-hand page write 'I need help with...' and write down all the things that don't feel quite in your control, or that you don't feel you manage as well as you could. So, depending on your circumstances, this list might include what you eat, when you sleep, where you go... write down what makes sense to you. Write down anything that makes your life difficult, whether it's directly related to surviving cancer or not, because if you're expending energy on struggling with it, you're using energy that could be helping you in your journey towards thriving.

When you have this list, on the right-hand page write 'Sources of help' and, for each area, note some ideas about where you could get help from. For example, if you've written 'I need help with finding more time to rest,' the right-hand page might say, 'Someone else cooks three nights a week' or 'I work from home one day per week' or 'Stop going to... (something you don't really enjoy but have got into the habit of doing)'.

Then do something with these plans. Talk to people, write reminders and stick them on the fridge, make appointments, whatever it takes to get you the help you need.

🌾 🌾 🌾

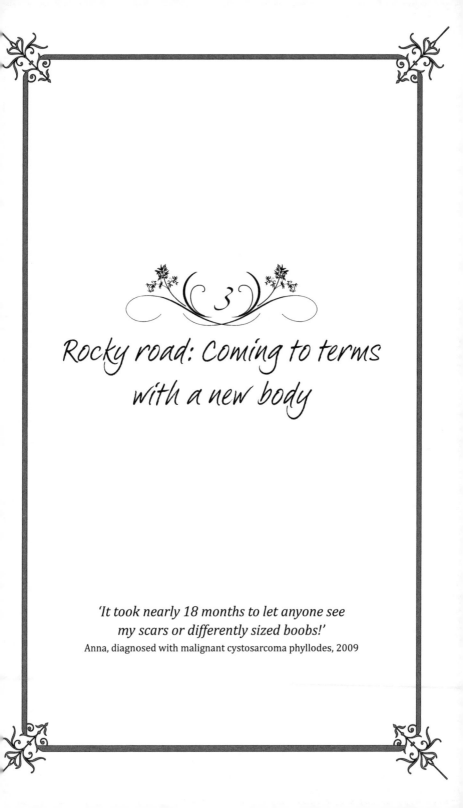

3

Rocky road: Coming to terms with a new body

'It took nearly 18 months to let anyone see my scars or differently sized boobs!'
Anna, diagnosed with malignant cystosarcoma phyllodes, 2009

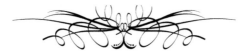

Not long after I was diagnosed – in fact, it must have been within the first few days, because I spent a fortnight before surgery trying to find The Perfect Pyjamas – I wondered whether cancer would make me stop caring about what I looked like.

I've always liked to look good – 'good' in this case meaning 'making the most of what I've got' rather than 'I'm just off to do some more modelling for Gucci' – and I've always made an effort. I own far too many shoes and dresses, and have stores of lipgloss that reach beyond any reasonable life expectancy. My hair gets a good cut every six weeks (apart from the bald bit at the beginning of 2009, for which I had a range of pretty hats, matched to my outfits) and my nails and eyebrows are usually in good order.

I know not everyone is like me. Cheese sauce on one of my trouser legs? Well, the other one's clean. Skirt and blouse don't match? Well, actually they do, as they're both floral. Hair in an elastic band dropped on the path by the postman, and why would you need more than two pairs of shoes? I've always envied these people, a bit. I've thought about how much simpler life must be if you don't much care what you look like, over and above being clean and tidy. I've imagined that these people must be full of confidence and strength, because they have no need to hide behind heels and highlights the way I do. I wondered whether cancer would cure me of my superficial attitude to the way I look.

Well, it didn't. I still can't get through an airport without buying a new mascara, to keep all of my other tubes of mascara company. And I'm a little bit sad about that, and a little bit pleased.

Chances are, you'll feel not-unwell in your head before you feel not-unwell in your body. Cancer treatment represents a major physical trauma in almost every respect. I haven't met anyone who's been through cancer who doesn't feel that they have a very different body coming out of the other end of it. Whether they've had minor surgery, a lung removed or a double mastectomy, there's a sense of newness. Sometimes it's a strong sense of mutilation, sometimes a fresh respect for what the body can survive, sometimes the idea of a gulf having opened up between the self and the body: cancer has divided me from myself.

But when you think about what needs to happen during treatment for cancer, it's hardly surprising that our relationships with our bodies change.

Coming up is a list of the physical collateral damage that came about as a result of my dance with cancer. Score one point for every one you can match, and a bonus for any that you have and I don't. We can compare notes in the bar later.

1. I have scars, lumps and puckering on my right breast where the tumour was removed. There's an area where there is no feeling at all, and another about half a centimetre away from the numb bit that is hypersensitive to touch and heat and cold, and sometimes feels as though it is gnawing at me. (With my largely-half-remembered-from-A-Level-Biology-not-quite-knowledge, I imagine that when I was stitched up again, all of the nerve endings got bunched together in one place, instead of being evenly distributed like they were before.)

2. I have two overlapping crescent scars and a crater in my right armpit where lymph nodes were taken to check for cancer spreading around my body. This check was carried out while I was on the operating table: the nodes were taken to Pathology – I like to think of them being transported by a roller-skating scrub nurse making a 'nee-nah' noise, but the journey was probably a little more prosaic than that – and examined while the surgery team got on with the rest of the cutting and removing and sewing up. Then the results meant that the rest of the lymph nodes got to stay in their natural habitat, rather than being removed. The armpit scars are still a little angrier than the others, but that might have been because one morning about a month after surgery I had a moment in the shower

when I forgot, for a minute, about the whole cancer thing, shaved my armpits, and took the scar tissue clean off with the razor.

3. I have a scar on my left breast where some possibly-cancerous-but-not-in-the-end-as-it-turned-out-thank-goodness cells were taken out. I resent and dislike this scar more than I do the right breast and lymph node ones. I think it must be because it turned out to be unnecessary. I see the other scars as part of the process that got me to wellness and recovery. This one feels like a needless mutilation. Also, it itches.

4. I lost all of my hair. Head. Eyebrows. Eyelashes. Armpits. Body hair. Pubic hair. The lot. It went quickly: over the course of about a week, I went from being fully tonsured in all respects, to bald and Brazilian. Well, not completely bald, ever. There were a few short wisps that clung on to the top of my head, making me look a bit like a gently rotting mushroom found at the back of the fridge, and allowing my family and friends to constantly exclaim that it was 'Definitely growing back. Definitely! It's longer than it was on Monday, for sure!' (I think we had one of those group hallucinations, like when 700 strangers from all over the world phone their local police to report having seen Marilyn Monroe eating cheese and juggling in the street.) It's certainly true that, if my hair had grown back at the rate we all believed it was growing, I'd have been able to shear it once a fortnight and knit enough jackets for an army battalion out of it. It all grew back in time. My eyebrows and lashes are much the same as they were before. Body hair is, I think, a little finer and more sparse. The hair on my head is thicker and the kink

at the front, which had been a law unto itself for as long as I could remember, didn't make it back. I am much, much more grey than I was before, but it's two years later, so I might have been anyway.

5. My teeth were damaged by the chemotherapy drugs. And how. Bits broke off. I had toothache for months. My gums bled at the very thought of a toothbrush – I had to resort to cleaning them with toothpaste on my finger at one stage. One of the chemotherapy nurses told me at the outset of treatment that I wasn't allowed to use a mouthwash because 'Mouthwash is meant for a healthy mouth and, once you start chemotherapy, your mouth won't be healthy.' She sure was right. At the time of writing, more than two years after chemotherapy finished, I'm still using the softest possible toothbrush, and listen to my husband's electric toothbrush whirring away with the envy that a 15-year-old aspiring motorcyclist on a pushbike must feel as a Harley-Davidson roars by. I carried a flask of hot salty water everywhere I went and rinsed my mouth every time I'd eaten. I took painkillers constantly. I had several abortive trips to the dentist and the dentistry department at the hospital, during which everyone agreed that intervention wasn't possible because of the risks involved in treating a chemotherapy patient. Chemotherapy drugs wipe out the immune system, so any exposure to infection must be avoided: no dental surgery, no going on the Tube, no kissing anyone who has a cold. Not that any of those are particular hardships, unless you've been up all night with a toothache. Also, there's a risk when having chemotherapy that once you start bleeding you won't stop, because the composition of the blood is different.

6. My mouth is still sore. (Also chemotherapy drugs.) Over the years the soreness has decreased from proper pain to constant tenderness, the way your arm feels after you bump it but before the bruise actually appears. I imagine that one day I'll wake up and spend the morning feeling a little bit disorientated, like when you dream it's Christmas Eve and, even though it's actually August, you spend your first few waking hours beating back the desire to peel Brussels sprouts and light the fire. Eventually I'll realize that the funny feeling is down to the fact that my mouth isn't hurting any more.

7. I have Irritable Bowel Syndrome. My gut never recovered from – you guessed it – the chemotherapy drugs, which kill all of the lovely friendly bacteria that line the human gut. (They're also in the mouth, hence point 6.) This means that it's difficult for the body to process food properly. During chemotherapy treatment, it's de rigueur to have chronic diarrhoea, but afterwards I find I have a digestive system that's a little bit wary of dairy produce, almost all fruit, sweet things, gluten and rich foods. I can eat all of these things occasionally and in moderation, but stomach pain, wind and diarrhoea are easily triggered by having a little too much of any of them. As someone who has spent most of her life eating pretty much anything (barring shellfish and bananas) with great enthusiasm, I find IBS tedious and annoying.

8. My nails are not in a good way. I was delighted – and lucky, given the state they were in – not to lose any nails during treatment, but they are still bad enough to make a manicurist blanch and go to get special basecoats called things like 'Super Iron Repair Daily Extra Strength' out of

the Problem Nails Drawer. My nails have stopped splitting vertically, something which is just ridiculously painful (a) because it tears at the flesh and (b) because, unless you are someone whose job and life involve sitting very still or wearing silk-lined gauntlets, it's really easy to catch, and tear, those splits a little bit more. Now they only split and flake horizontally, which is manageable. My nails are now what I can truly say is a healthy pink at the base, the colour of the insides of those tiny shells you find every step or so on the shore after a high tide, but by the time they get to the tip they have become a jaundiced yellow flecked with white. I keep thinking I'm on the brink of a French manicure, but never quite make it.

9. The inside of my nose is permanently dry. It bleeds if I forget to put Vaseline up there; I have a sleek two-fingered coating action now that I should probably patent, or teach.

10. I have two sets of scars on my left arm from the PICC (Peripherally Inserted Central Catheter). Each is a trio of marks: one from the place where the line went in, two more from the stitches that held the external hardware in place. Essentially, I look as though I could plug two three-pin plugs into my arm. I don't mind these too much. Partly because I've never had the sort of arms that make a career of T-shirt-and-bracelet-modelling likely, and partly because the scars are about a thousand times better than having the actual line in.

11. I have a little blue tattoo between my breasts and another halfway down my right side – a gift from the radiotherapy people to allow them to line the beams up correctly.

These I resent. They are exactly the sort of thing that is chucked in at the end of conversations, and done with a minimum of fuss and preamble, along with, 'Sorry for the scratch' (subtext: 'You've had much bigger needles with much nastier stuff poked into you, so please don't make a fuss, because I'm going to do this anyway, and it's For Your Own Good.'). The little blue dot on my side isn't really an issue – midriff tops and I have never really been on so much as nodding terms – but the one between my breasts… grrrr. I look as though I dropped a pen down my cleavage. From time to time I wonder about using the pesky blue dot as the starting point for a tattoo – maybe a heart or a flower, or even a little dragon – but, to be honest, I'm pretty much over needles for now.

12. My right breast (the radiotherapied one) appears suntanned, and is a different colour to the surrounding skin. My right nipple, conversely, is paler than my left one, so my breasts appear as though one is the photographic negative of the other. Like the PICC scars, this doesn't bother me a great deal, because 40 is a bit late in the day to be starting a topless modelling career, and because when you've had a breast cancer diagnosis, having any breasts at all at the end of treatment is, quite frankly, a bonus.

13. I am undergoing a medical menopause, which means several big physical changes. Obviously, my periods have stopped. (Well, they stopped during chemotherapy, and the drugs I take now just keep them stopped.) My skin is as dry as paper and as thirsty as a rose bush in a heat wave. I've declined to put on weight – I refuse to do so just because the leaflet in a box of tablets tells me

to – but the extra weight I do have has somehow shifted around my body and got comfortable on my upper arms and stomach. (OK, maybe it hasn't actually moved. Maybe I've actually lost a bit of weight, but not from those places. I will agree that, technically, that's more likely. But I swear that there are times when I feel that, if I looked in the mirror quickly enough, I'd see little pouches of fat making their way from place to place, shifting under my skin like knees under a blanket.)

14. I have permanently swollen feet and hands. It's not dramatic: they haven't taken on the appearance of medical gloves blown up and tied at the wrist by over-excited medical students during Freshers' Week. (Apart from during the overweight and too-hot summer following chemotherapy.) My hands and feet have just, well, gone up a size. My wedding and engagement rings had to be cut off and we had a new wedding ring made, because the difference in size was too great to get the old one adjusted.

15. Cramp. Aaaaaargh, the cramp. It started during chemotherapy. Essential trace elements like potassium and magnesium get used up as the body tries to cope with the onslaught it's under, and the gut isn't capable, in its depleted state, of absorbing more. And the lack of those trace elements – coupled with the fact that muscles probably aren't being used as much as they are used to – means cramp. Now, two years on, it's not so bad. It's 'Ow!' cramp. It's cramp that I can almost sleep through. There was a time, though, when cramp catapulted me out of bed in the middle of the night. I cried. I screamed. I shook. I'm pretty sure I freaked out the neighbourhood cats, and I don't think my family

liked it much, either. Thank heavens for quinine tablets, and time. I'm still lucky to get through 24 hours without something cramping somewhere, though.

So there you are. As a result of cancer, I have a body affected for the worse in almost every way. And yes, I am still alive, and yes, I am grateful, and yes, I am still me, and I can still do most of what I want to do, including going out into the world and being unremarkable in a crowd, because I'm not obviously disfigured by my dance with cancer. (At least not from a distance.) But I found that coming to terms with the changes in my body was a hard thing to do. For a while it was as though my body was that old friend who went off on a round-the-world trip and came back a person I just couldn't feel comfortable with again, no matter how much time I spent trying.

Eventually, I worked out that what I needed to do was to focus on, and deal with, the changes rather than having a sense of otherness and a list of grumbles, which is what I walked around with for months. It's not the most comfortable process, but it's one that I think was worthwhile, and one that I've used with some other people who have found it helpful, too.

BAH! THINKING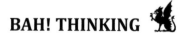

Taking an inventory

Take a pen and paper and find a quiet spot near a mirror.

Start by thinking about the part(s) of your body where the cancer was. Take a look at them. Look at the scars. Run your fingers over them. Look at the colour, the shape, what they do to the skin around them. Think about the feel of them. Examine them, thoroughly, until they stop being a part of you and become something abstract, like a blown-up image of a fruit fly or a photograph of skin so magnified it appears more like a desert landscape than the back of someone's hand.

Write down the scars. Itemize them. What shape, colour, position are they? What do they remind you of?

Next, look at, and think about, all of the outside of your body. It might help to start at your head and work down, or your feet and work up. Write down every change that's occurred due to cancer: hair, skin, changes to nails, whatever they are.

Now turn your attention to what's within. Again, it might help to start at one end of you and mentally scan your way to the other. What's damaged, or just different, inside you? Write those changes down.

Remember, you're not writing a list of all the ways in which you differ from a supermodel, or of all of the bits of you that you don't much like, or what's changed since you were 17. Only the changes cancer has wrought in your body.

So, now you have a list.

Take a moment to read through the list, and to acknowledge that that's a lot of changes.

When you're ready – and it might be immediately, or it might be that you need to give yourself a bit of time to let the effects of having taken a direct look at your body wear off, especially if you haven't really taken a close inventory before – it's time to work out what changes matter enough to do something about them. So, when you're ready, move on to the next thinking session. If you don't feel up to it yet, skip ahead and come back to it when you do. This book isn't the boss of you; it will wait for you.

BAH! THINKING 🦅
The body change scorecard

For each item on the list, write down how much the change bugs you, '1' being 'I barely notice it' and '10' being 'I think about it all the time.' (Anything scoring 5 or below should be, essentially, livable-with.) Do this without too much thought: your first instinct is probably correct here.

When you are done, take a look at those physical changes that rate from 6 to 10. These are the changes that you find difficult to bear: the ones that cause you some mental and/or physical discomfort on a regular basis. These are the changes that you need to do something about. You didn't survive cancer, my friend, to have your life blighted by the fall-out from it. And suffering in silence is not really good for you – not for your body, your heart or your life.

For each item on your list, ask yourself, 'Why is this a problem?' (You might want to get someone else to help you with this.) Challenge yourself. If you're not talking to someone, you could write the 'conversation' you're having with yourself down. For example:

My scars are a 7.

Why are they a problem?

Because they are ugly.

What's ugly about them?

They just look horrible.

OK. Why do they look horrible?

Because when I look at them I think of cancer.

Is there anything else about them?

They remind me of a horrible time.

Why was it horrible?

Because I was frightened. Because I was so ill. Because I might have died.

So, now we know why the scars are a 7: because of what they stand for as much as what they look like.

The next stage is to find a new way to think about those scars. For example, you might think that instead of seeing them as a reminder that you might have died, you could see them as a symbol of the fact that you are alive. (That you are thriving, even.) Write that down, too. Something like:

'My scars are a sign that I am now thriving,' or 'Scars mean I'm alive' or 'These scars mean that I am well.'

This is your new thought about the area that's causing you problems.

Every time you catch yourself thinking about your scars, examining them, looking for them in a mirror – every time you find that your fingers have, without permission, drifted to where your scars lie (I'm fairly sure that if I wasn't a two-handed typist and a spare-time knitter I'd spend most of my time unaware that I had one hand down my top, fingers running absently over the puckers, dips and pleats that remain) – stop and think, deliberately, whatever your replacement thought is: 'My scars are a sign that I am now thriving.' Say it out loud if it helps. Say it to a mirror if it helps. (Looking in a mirror helps me to absorb the words better. I'm not sure why.) The important thing is to do it every time that old thought comes to mind.

Do this consistently for a week, and then ask yourself what the score for this symptom is now. It should have reduced dramatically.

Do this consistently for a fortnight, and it will have become second nature. Check the score again. It should still be dropping.

A bit of judiciously applied Bah! thinking can work wonders when you need to come to terms with some of the changes that cancer brings to your body. But it isn't magic thinking dust; a sprinkle of different thinking won't make everything better. For example, I gained weight during chemotherapy, and every time I couldn't get my jeans over my backside I was thoroughly upset and annoyed by the extra slabs of myself that had wobbled on. (Which was every morning, pretty much, because I always hoped yesterday was a temporary error made by my trousers, rather than the cumulative effect of all the custard and rice pudding and ice-cream I ate to keep the heartburn and sickness at bay, and all of the biscuits and chocolates I ate because people kept bringing them when they dropped in to see how I was doing.) I could have looked myself in the eye, said 'I am the size I was before chemotherapy,' put on some used-to-be-too-big trousers and gone to have a thick slice of that leftover chocolate fudge cake for breakfast.

It wouldn't have helped a bit.

Part of the business of thriving is the business of taking responsibility.

BLOG POST, 7 MARCH 2011 (ABRIDGED): MWAHAHAHAHA

That, my friends, is the sound of my arch-enemy, Captain Cramp. Yes, he's back, with his evil laugh and his shiny spurs and his frankly ridiculous moustache. He's mainly going for my left hamstring, but occasionally the hamstring and calf. From 5 a.m. onwards he goes for the arch of my foot and I can't work out how to stretch it out when I'm still quite asleep, so I just spend a couple of hours drifting and feeling uncomfortable. In a completely new and worrying development, my right shoulder has been cramping too.

But, I have a plan.

1. I will keep drinking my daily tonic water. Sometimes with gin.

2. I will go to my GP and get some quinine tablets, which are absolutely brilliant. You're supposed to take them as a preventative measure, but I sometimes forget and end up taking them during a cramp attack. It's like pouring water onto the Wicked Witch of the West. The cramp just melts away. Magic.

3. I will start taking magnesium and potassium tissue salts again.

4. Although I make sure I take some exercise every day, I'll start doing a regular yoga and Pilates class again, so I can start getting stronger.

But here's the most important thing I'm going to do.

5. I'm going to remember that I need to look after myself all the time, rather than letting things slide when I feel well and so allowing Captain Cramp to sneak back into my life. Oh yes I am. So, Captain Cramp, make the most of it while you can, because you won't be here for long.

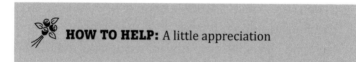 **HOW TO HELP:** A little appreciation

It's obvious, of course, that no matter what physical changes cancer has wrought on your beloved/friend/sister/father – weight gain, weight loss, strange new hair, scars, ageing, teeth like an explosion in a granite factory – you love them just the same. It's obvious that their changed appearance won't make a bit of difference to you.

It's obvious. That doesn't mean it should go without saying.

The long trek to thriving might mean regaining self-esteem and putting a lot of time and effort into accepting a new body, and/or regaining elements of the old one. It would be lovely if you could notice, and comment on, either the bits that have never changed or the bits that are, as it were, under review.

******

We've spent a lot of time thinking about the collateral damage that cancer has caused. But what about what *hasn't* changed? Here's my list.

- Somehow, I still have nice breasts. Not the kind of breasts that will ever be paid millions to model a bikini, you understand, but in a good bra and a well-cut top I have a bosom to be proud of. A bosom that, occasionally, gets an admiring second glance.

- I still have the knees of a footballer. (Not the talent, or the stamina, or the fitness or the bank balance, though.)

- I have ears that are fundamentally incompatible with earbud speakers. Those cute little buds just will not stay in, and I regularly have ear envy when I see other people wearing them. Of course, breast cancer treatment wasn't going to change the shape of my ear canal, I know that. But it amuses me that every time I buy something that comes with earbuds, I try them and get annoyed when they fall out. And I like that I was doing this waaaay before cancer, and I'm still doing it now. It reminds me that the body I had was one that I wasn't universally appreciative of, so there's no reason why I have to expect perfection now.

- For all of the pain that's going on inside my mouth most of the time, I have the same smile, and when I smile it, it still works: it still says what I want it to say. (Someone told me that when I smile I look 'the way I always had and always will', and that was something that helped me no end during rueful reflections on my menopausal skin and chemotherapy-sized backside.)

- If you ignore all of the menopausal crow's feet that are going on, my eyes are the same as they always were, common-or-garden blue; but when I focus on them in my reflection, I can look at the person I was before my dance with cancer began, and recognize the one still to come, when thriving is such second nature that I barely notice that I'm doing it.

What's on your list?

Travelling companions:
The more, the merrier

*'I've learned that some friends and family
will astound you with kindness and
thoughtfulness and some will astound you
with thoughtlessness.'*

Debbie, diagnosed with anal cancer in 2011

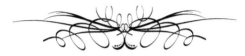

BLOG POST, 7 NOVEMBER 2011:
FOR THOSE WHO CARE

We all know that life's not unrelentingly wonderful. Of course it isn't. But right now, I seem to know, or know of, a lot of people who are seriously ill, and even more who are supporting those people, trying to get them well, trying to get them home, or simply trying to get them comfortable.

And it's reminded me of something that I've often thought about during my dance with cancer: it might be lousy out there on the dance floor, with bits of your body crumbling or crumpling, with your sudden inability to do the simplest things, like sleep and eat and breathe, with the way your life has to stop in its tracks while you are forced to do this lousy thing you didn't ever ask for, but I still think it has to be better than watching someone you love do it.

All the time I was ill, I fully understood what was happening in my body, or at least I fully understood the sensations. I knew exactly where I was in my mind. Somewhere deep inside me I felt strong and safe in the world, even though all hell was breaking loose in my breasts and bowels and sleeping patterns because of cancer and cancer treatment. I was sure that I wouldn't die. I was clear that I was managing. I felt, somehow, alright despite it all. (Except when I didn't. But even then, at least I had a full understanding of what was happening.)

But I couldn't always communicate that well enough. Despite all of my blogging and talking and trying really hard to explain, I knew that the people around me were looking at me and wondering: was I as alright as I seemed? When I said I wasn't hungry, did it mean I wasn't hungry or was it a sign of something else: did they need to cajole me into eating or let me be? When I had a big cry, then dried my eyes, said I was all right, and picked up my knitting again, they had to figure out whether I really was OK. My family and friends had a lot to carry: the weight of watching someone they love undergo some fairly brutal treatment; the fact of not really being quite sure of anything; and somewhere, I imagine, the secret fear of wondering whether this was The Beginning Of The End. (I had that one too, but with the comfort that, if I was going to die, at least I wasn't going to have to live through me dying, if you see what I mean. Selfish, but true.)

So, if you are one of those people who, right now, are watching someone you love struggle – whether it's with cancer or MS or mental illness or depression or recovery from injury – then I have some things to say to you.

– I know your life must be really difficult right now. It's OK for you to know that too. Yes, you just have to get on with it, but you can also say – to yourself, or to others – that you are having a difficult time. Just because you don't have The Thing, doesn't mean you aren't affected by The Thing.

– The person you are caring for might be in too much pain or distress or drug-related stuff to express it, but somewhere in there they know you're there and they appreciate what you're doing.

– You're allowed to share the burden. You're allowed to take the day off and ask someone else to make the hospital visit/take the meal/do the shopping.

– Please take care of you. You're precious and important too.

– Remember that if you're doing the best that you can do, that's good enough. Even if it does mean sometimes getting a bit tetchy and tearful and frustrated. That's part of being human, and your humanity is what's doing all of the work here.

– Thank you. I might not know you, but I appreciate what you're doing.

And here's a tip that you can take or leave. One of the hardest things about a Big Thing Going Wrong is that it's easy for everyone to be so busy dealing with the Big Thing that the person gets a little bit forgotten. So, before you next see the person that you're caring for, think about them before this crisis hit. Think of the things they did, the way they were, the time you shared. And use those memories as the basis for the way you treat them. You'll both be glad of it.

******

When I moved back to Northumberland, after 20 years in London, one of the unexpected best things about it was the fact that I got to be ordinary again. Me popping in for a cup of tea was no longer a thrice-annual (if that) occasion. I got to see friends and say goodbye to them without great ceremony, because we both knew that we'd probably bump into each other again before the week was out. Of course it was fun to be a Special Occasion, and to spend my limited time in Northumberland like a minor royal. But I much prefer my new everydayness. And it's not unlike the feeling I started to get when I was first on the road to thriving.

Don't get me wrong: I appreciated everything that the people around me did for me when I was unwell. But what I appreciated even more was hitting the point where special consideration was no longer necessary. We didn't need to eat out in restaurants close to my home to protect me from late nights and germy trains. I was included in group 'who wants to get together?' emails, rather than being consulted in advance. I could go out for coffee and never mention cancer, because there were more immediate and interesting things to discuss.

This was lovely for me. I wouldn't say that my friendships and family relationships were 'back to normal', because cancer changed them all. They became, for the most part, richer, deeper, stronger. And once I had learned, via my dance with cancer, that I didn't have to do everything on my own, I think I became better at relationships because I was able to be more honest about what was happening in my life. So, things didn't go back to normal. But I did get to be one of the crowd again.

And then the conversations started. Over lunch, a friend told me about the first time her mother had cancer, and how frightened she had been, and how my experience had brought all that back. A colleague told me how supporting me had helped her to forgive herself for not doing more when a friend of hers was dying. Family members talked me through how they had felt when I was diagnosed, ill, recovering, ill again, in a way they never had at the time. And I thought: these people – all the people who watch as we dance with cancer – deserve more credit and help than they get.

BAH! THINKING 🐉
Making it better

There is a kind of logic to the fact that the point at which you are ready to stop talking and thinking about cancer is the time the people around you need to start. Here are some ideas to help them.

- *Unless it will really distress you to continue the conversation, allow your friends, family and loved ones to talk about what happened when you were ill. My mother came with me to one of my chemotherapy sessions, and was helpful and kind and matter-of-fact about the whole thing. Afterwards, she told my husband that she 'hadn't liked seeing all that stuff go in'. The least I can do now is talk about cancer when she wants to talk about it.*

- *Say thank you. Say it in a genuine way, and put some effort into the way you say it. Write letters, send cards, sing songs, compose poetry, pick up the phone, grow cuttings from the rose bush someone sent you when you came out of hospital and give them away, knit socks (again, probably just me). The best way to say thank you is to be specific: 'I appreciated everything you did for me when I was ill, but especially the way you always remembered I got upset the day before treatment, and called or came round.'*

- *Make the effort to show people that you are ready to be a full part of their lives again. Whether they realize it or not, some of the people who love you will be protecting you from what's going on for them, so you need to take the initiative and meet them more than halfway. If you know that someone in your life is having difficulty, reach out. Email with a specific offer of help, call at a time when you know they will be able to talk, focus on them.*

• *Organize something meaningful for you and the people who have supported you to do. You could take part in a walk to raise money for a cancer charity, paint a room at a hospice, fundraise to provide something that you all agree would have made your dance with cancer easier. (Like reclining chemotherapy chairs that actually recline, and aren't covered with that nasty plastic that makes you sweat.) It's an opportunity for everyone to channel their feelings into positive action. And when so many people feel so helpless watching us dance with cancer, that's a great thing.*

• *Be yourself. I think I went a bit 'eyes and teeth' for a while, like an unknown actress who has somehow got down to the last two to play Elizabeth Taylor in a film directed by Spielberg. I really wanted to show everyone that I was fine, so they could stop worrying. Of course, the reverse happened. They sensed my lack of authenticity and wondered what I was hiding. Relax. Be. Smile. But only if you feel like smiling.*

I have given up trying to work out what my family would be like if cancer hadn't shown up in my life. Obviously it's a pointless exercise anyway, like attempting to decide whether your hangover was caused by the gin or the wine, or whether you've got a headache because you always get a headache when the weather's like this. But that didn't stop me from spending months thinking about the impact cancer had had. Did Alan look tired because of all the emotional strain we had been through? Did we love each other more, or would we have been this close anyway? Were Ned and Joy more confident or less confident, happier or sadder than they would have been if life had been more ordinary? (For 'ordinary' read 'perfect' in my thinking: sadly, there's nothing extraordinary about having a cancer.)

BAH! THINKING

Moving relationships on

Find a quiet place. Take your notebook with you.

First, make a list of everyone you think helped to 'love you better'. (I know it's not really as simple as love making you better. I also know that, if you didn't have people to love you, survival might well be possible, but thriving would be a non-starter.)

Then think about every person in turn. Think about what they've done for you, and think about how your relationship is now. Do you need to thank them? Is there something you'd like to resolve, or check out, or discuss? Or is your relationship healthy? Write down what you need to do. If you want to, thank them, to yourself in your heart or out loud. Take a moment to appreciate that person.

Then move on to the next person on your list.

You don't have to do everyone at once. Your people, your rules. Do this the way you feel comfortable: one a day, just before the next time you see a particular person, in writing, in your head.

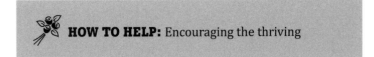

HOW TO HELP: Encouraging the thriving

- Let your newly thriving loved one help you. Tell them what you're worried about, ask their advice, ring them for a rant after a lousy day.

- By all means be kind and compassionate, but leave your kid gloves at home. Trust your loved one to tell you if they're tired or sad or want to go home.

- Be honest about what effect watching your loved one dance with cancer has had on you. Tell them you felt frightened, or overawed, or helpless, or all three.

- Remember what the basis of your relationship is, and act accordingly. I have a few friends that I've met via cancer, but many more friendships have been forged in knitting shops, over dinner, on trips to the theatre or while searching for the shoes that one of us has in our head. Go back to that basis: suggest that you do something that you used to do, not in a nostalgic 'let's go back to the place we were before cancer came along' way, but in the spirit of whatever it was that made you friends in the first place.

- And keep doing whatever it is that you've been doing, because if you are close enough to someone who has danced with cancer to be reading this book, you've got a lot right.

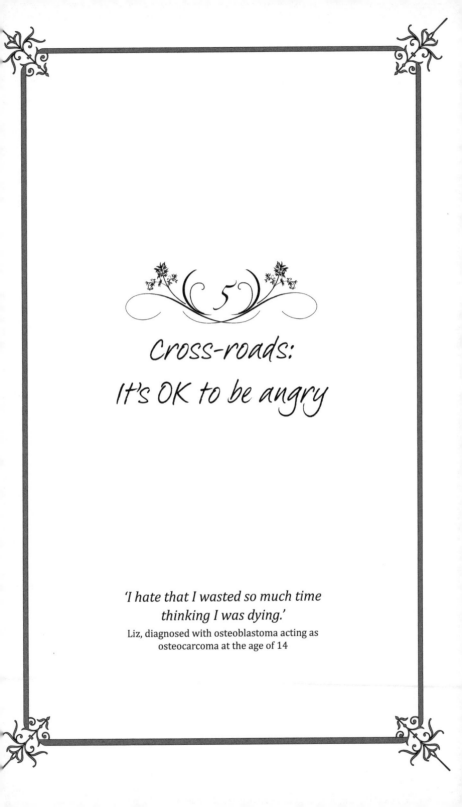

5

Cross-roads:
It's OK to be angry

*'I hate that I wasted so much time
thinking I was dying.'*
Liz, diagnosed with osteoblastoma acting as
osteocarcoma at the age of 14

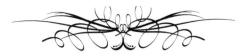

don't think of myself as being angry. I don't slam doors or shout. I don't like arguments and I get uncomfortable around people who rage and storm. I was driving my daughter somewhere recently when someone pulled out in front of me and I had to put the brakes on to avoid running into the back of them. 'I don't think you really had time to do that, did you?' I muttered in the direction of the other driver. 'That was you doing road rage, wasn't it, Mum?' Joy said, and she was right. Anger and me don't really go. Or that's what I'd like to think.

BLOG POST, 26 JANUARY 2012 (EXCERPT): BESIDE MYSELF

OK, I thought, I'm not someone who is angry about cancer. There was a corner of me feeling a little bit smug. Too well-adjusted to get mad, it whispered, don't you worry about it. But in another corner, another voice was whispering too. I didn't think I was going to like what it had to say, so I ignored it for as long as I could. But in the end I gave in and listened.

The voice was saying, 'You are angry, but you can't admit it, so you let it out in different ways.' And as soon as I listened, that smugness disappeared in a puff of… whatever imaginary voices in hypothetical corners of the psyche disappear into. (You know what they say: every analogy limps.) Because all of those cleverly-written-so-you-don't-realize-quite-how-ranty-they-are rants about hospital waiting times, rude oncologists, scars, PICCs, not being able to work, breathe, do what I want to do? Anger. Anger at the fact that I got a cancer, redirected at things it felt OK to be annoyed about.

I suppose my feelings are further complicated by the fact that, nasty as cancer is, my life has been improved a great deal by my dance with it. So being angry about cancer has felt a bit like being angry with the teacher who pushed you and pushed you… until you got full marks in your exam.

But maybe it's time to admit that I was angry that I got a cancer. Yes, I laughed and I danced, but actually, getting a cancer really hacked me off. It ruined my plans. It upset my family. It turned me fat and bald and knackered. It hurt. And I didn't rage and scream, because I'm not a rager and a screamer – Bah! is about as cross as I get – but I was angry all the same.

I don't think I'm angry any more. But if cancer ever comes back to me… I'll be mad as all hell. And I won't be afraid to say so.

BAH! THINKING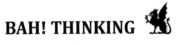

Recognizing anger

Anger takes a lot of different forms. Take a few moments to think about the way you show anger. You might be a straight-out-of-the-movies, bricks-through-windows type, but most of us aren't. Do you recognize any of these expressions of anger?

- *Long, theatrical sighs*

- *Tearfulness*

- *Out-of-proportion annoyance at something trivial*

- *Dreams full of arguments, shouting and fury*

- *Doing things with too much force: not realizing that you've slammed a door until you jump, or banging a coffee down until it's spilled*

- *Sarcasm*

- *Being unable to let arguments go*

If any, or all, of these behaviours feel as though they are taking up a disproportionate amount of time in your life, it's probably a good time to admit that you are angry. And it's OK to be angry. If you've been through cancer, and cancer treatment, angry is a reasonable place to be. Remember, just because you're alive, you're not now morally obliged to skip around scattering rose petals for the rest of your days.

The trick with anger – I am, eventually, learning – is not to try not to have it, but to let it out at the right place, in the right time. Otherwise… well. Let me tell you about something I've been ashamed of since it happened.

I was at oncology clinic. I'd waited for a long time. I was waiting for a check-up, the point of which was to declare me well enough to have chemotherapy a couple of days later. ('Well enough', in oncology terms, means enough white blood cells to indicate that the unseen but essential bits of your body, the bone marrow and the blood, are recovered enough from the last onslaught to survive another one. So you can be a whey-faced, vomiting, weeping wreck and still 'well'. Oncology is an odd planet: I suspect that the expression 'kill or cure' originated there.)

So, the system was: check-up on Monday, and if you are 'well' enough, treatment on Wednesday. I think I was waiting for the all-clear for my fourth round, so I was tetchy and tearful, and in possession of a couple more chins than I'd had at the beginning of chemotherapy, something that I wasn't happy about at all. In short, I was not in a place you'd want to go to on holiday.

While I was waiting to be seen, one of the Macmillan nurses came to talk to me about the next treatment. We had a bit of a prickly relationship – she thought my decision to keep working when I could during treatment was bloody-mindedness, and I thought her desire to make all patients conform to her ideas about What Was Best disrespectful. I'd scheduled the work that I was doing around the chemotherapy cycle: I didn't work during treatment week, as I would be feeling the ill-effects; I didn't work in the second week, as my immune system was flat on the floor that week so I stayed close to home; but I worked the third week. Because I'm self-employed (and with expensive tastes), I had to work when I could. Because I'm a specialist I tend to get booked up in advance. Because I was determined to stay professional I refused to change plans with my clients unless things went drastically wrong. (This wasn't new. Before cancer came along, I once ran a day of training while in the grip of food poisoning. Memorable for everyone, and not in a good way.) I'm not saying that my work ethic was a good one: I'm just telling you how it was.

'Stephanie,' the nurse breezed at me, 'your next cycle is the week of a bank holiday, so there's no clinic on the Monday, so treatment will need to be delayed by a week, OK?'

'I'm working away that week,' I said. 'Could we do the chemo on the Thursday or the Friday of the week it's scheduled for at the moment?' I didn't mind making it another day. I knew the chemotherapy unit operated every day. The nurse rolled her eyes. 'We did warn you,' she said, unnecessarily patiently and with a smile that was anything but a smile, 'that you need to be flexible with your treatment.'

And I had been warned. I'd been warned that if my bloodwork results weren't good enough, if I had a cold, if I was unwell, then I would have to defer my treatment. And if that had happened, I'd have been a good grown-up and explained to my clients that I needed to move or cancel the session, because my health came first on this occasion. But lose two days of paid work that I desperately needed because the oncology clinic couldn't manoeuvre itself round one bank holiday?

No. Not OK. I think this was one of the only times in my life that I've felt truly, incandescently angry.

And I shouted to the back of the retreating nurse, 'I do have a life, you know.' And ever since, I've wished I hadn't. Other people in the waiting room tutted and shook their heads. The nurse rolled her eyes in the most long-suffering manner imaginable.

To be fair to me, it was the culmination of months of frustration. It was the final straw.

But what I don't like about this outburst – and, by extension, about 'proper' anger – is that it didn't really do justice to how I was feeling. I rolled up sadness, fear, frustration, the feeling that my life was out of my control, the aches in my bones, the baldness, the scars, the fat and I let them come out of me in a sentence of childish stroppiness. And I think that's why I control my anger: why I'm inclined to talk about things later, when I've chosen the words, when I've made myself as certain as I can be that I won't be misunderstood. Getting it wrong feels like a waste. I feel ashamed of the way I behaved that day, but actually I had a point. I just didn't express it very well, and I didn't express it to the right person.

BAH! THINKING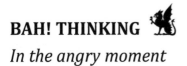
In the angry moment

Here are some good strategies for getting through a flare of anger (without annoying a nurse with the power to make your life even more of a misery – although, to give her credit, this one didn't). Depending on the situation, some will be more appropriate than others: a howl is probably not the best way to go into a meeting with your boss.

- *Breathe. I know it sounds ridiculous, but it really works. The fight-or-flight reflex encourages us to take a lot of shallow, quick breaths. Deliberate deep breathing slows down the anger reflex, and allows your brain to get the oxygen it needs to be able to think logically.*

- *Run, jump, hit something (soft and inanimate) or do some other physically strenuous activity that will help your body to redirect the energy that comes with anger.*

- *Shout. That's 'shout', not 'shout at': your shouting should direct anger away from the immediate situation. Growl, say 'aaargh', and do it until you feel the anger pass from your body. (If you watch a toddler have a tantrum, you'll see how they go limp afterwards. Your shout should empty the anger from you.)*

- *Focus intently on something. Look at your shoes and see what differences you can see between them. Try to remember the telephone numbers of everyone you know. Count the tiles on the ceiling, the lines on your palm, the number of objects in the room.*

Anger has a purpose. Anger is there to tell us that something is wrong, and that we need to act. Unfortunately, anger evolved – as part of our fight-or-flight mechanism – before higher brain function did, and so when we are angry we are incapable of logical, rational thought. The most constructive thing to do with anger is to listen to it. The problem is that, when we are angry – whether we are throwing teapots or sitting quietly while plotting an elaborate revenge – we can't hear what it is trying to say. So we need to find ways to get anger out of our systems, and then think about how we can deal with what made us angry.

BAH! THINKING

After the storm

Once the immediate storm, be it in the form of a yell, a sarcastic comment or an internal rant, has passed, it's time to discover what it is that anger is trying to tell you, and then do something about it.

- *Articulate the problem. Tell someone what happened and use them to help you identify what made you angry in that moment. Start a sentence with the words, 'What was behind the anger was...' without knowing what you are going to say next. Ask them what they think caused you to be angry. Listen to their response.*

- *If you prefer, write down what happened. But do the same thing: start a sentence with the words, 'What was behind the anger was...' and see what you write next.*

- *If you need to, apologize. The sooner, and the simpler, the better. 'I'm sorry I raised my voice. I was angry because I'd had to wait so long, but I shouldn't have taken it out on you.' 'I apologize for suggesting that you weren't a real doctor. I was feeling very frustrated because I didn't feel that you were taking my worries about whether I am really clear of cancer seriously, but there was no need for me to be rude.'*

- *Once you have identified the source of the anger, take action. If you burst into tears after a perfectly reasonable request from someone because you're tired – go to bed. If you're frustrated by the way your doctor talks to you at your check-up, ask to have a meeting with them to talk about how you'd prefer to be treated, or ask to be seen by another doctor in future. If you feel you have been treated badly, write a letter of complaint, calmly stating what you think went wrong and what you would like to be done differently in the future, whether for your own sake or for the sake of those trekking along the road to thriving behind you. But before you make the phone call or post the letter, make sure that you're not angry anymore, and check that what you're doing is proportionate, appropriate and in the right direction. (Just like I didn't when I shouted at that nurse.)*

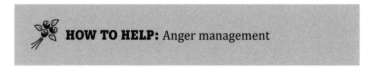

HOW TO HELP: Anger management

- Recognize that the moment, or hour, or day of rage is not the time to be able to have a sensible discussion about what is making your loved one angry. Wait until they are calm again.

- Allow your loved one to be angry. They probably have something to be angry about. It's tempting to rush in and solve it, I know, but don't. Let them rant and rave. Remember, as grandmothers everywhere say, 'Better out than in.'

- Be ready to talk about whatever is making your loved one angry. Rather than telling them what you think the problems are, ask them to tell you. Ask them whether they think they need help with understanding or resolving the issues they are angry about.

- Be prepared to recognize and act if things get out of control. Anger can be healthy; violence isn't. Crying and raging is a reasonable response in short bursts, but not for prolonged periods. If you're concerned, wait until a calm moment, then insist on getting some help.

- Remember that you, too, are entitled to be angry. You don't have to be A Rock all of the time. Cancer will have hurt and upset you, too, and 'just' because the damage is indirect doesn't mean you aren't allowed to feel strongly about it. Use the strategies in this chapter to help acknowledge and deal with your own anger.

🌱 🌱 🌱

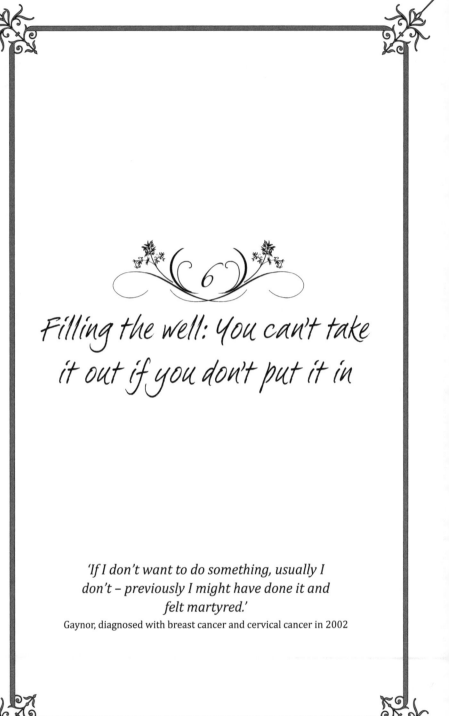

6

Filling the well: You can't take it out if you don't put it in

'If I don't want to do something, usually I don't – previously I might have done it and felt martyred.'
Gaynor, diagnosed with breast cancer and cervical cancer in 2002

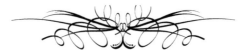

Many years ago, a friend told me about how she and her husband managed their relationship. They envisioned it, she said, as a lake. Whenever there were difficult times – sleepless nights with their spectacularly colicky newborn, arguments, no money in the bank, long work hours, illnesses – they saw themselves as drawing extra strength and sustenance from the lake in order to keep them going. That's nice, I said, thinking that I couldn't see how an analogy would help any relationship that was just-about-functioning on four hours of sleep a night thanks to a very unhappy baby. My friend got that I didn't get it. She explained that it only worked – they could only go to the lake and take from it – if they took the trouble to fill it. The crucial thing was adding to the lake. The mornings one of them got up and left the other sleeping, the dinner kept warm, the touches to the small of the back, the babysitter arranged, the odd why-don't-we-go-and-see-your-mother? and just-leave-that-I'll-do-it-in-the-morning… all of these small signs and gestures of love and care added to the lake and meant that there was something there when they needed to draw on it.

I never forgot this, and now Alan and I do a similar thing in our marriage – we talk about 'filling the well', and make a deliberate effort to make time for us and to be kind to each other. (And if you're thinking that, surely, people should be making time and being kind anyway, well, you're right, but a quick glance at the divorce statistics may convince you that a little well-filling is worth a try.)

My dance with cancer taught me something that I hadn't realized before, though.

You have to fill your own well. You have to nurture yourself.

I've met a lot of people who, during a dance with cancer, have felt truly let down by the people around them: the partners who have left, the children who have shrugged and turned away, the friends who have vanished like snow off a dyke. And these people are hurt. And that is completely understandable. But what they haven't seen, because they've been drawn to this area of betrayal in their lives the way the rest of your fingers can't leave a hangnail alone, is that the onus for looking after them doesn't only rest with the people around them. It rests with them, too.

And I don't think that the ability to nurture yourself is as important anywhere else as it is when it comes to this early part of the journey from survival to thriving. It makes the difference between someone permanently psychologically scarred by a dance with cancer, and someone who can say, 'Cancer? Yup, I had a cancer thing going on for a while. It wasn't pretty, but it's over.'

It's so, so easy to think that sometimes life is horrible because, you know, it's horrible, and bad things are happening because life's like that and there's nothing you can do, right? Well, no. (And if you're reading this book you probably already know that.) We can't always control what happens to us, but we can control how we respond, and that's where filling the well – having some resources to draw from – is important.

BAH! THINKING
Filling your own well

Find a quiet place and your notebook, and make a list of the things that you can do that nurture you and make you feel good. I find it helpful to have categories of things:

- *Easy, on-your-own things, like always having a 'to-read' pile/list of books to go to when you need one, or having a dog/having access to a dog that is always up for a good long walk, or subscribing to a magazine that you then put to one side for when you need it. (I do that with Private Eye, because it always makes me laugh and laugh.)*

- *Easy, free things, like taking a bath in the afternoon or sorting out a little pile of old DVDs that you'd love to watch again.*

- *Hobbies. I know they are a bit unfashionable, but having something that you love to do can be a lifesaver. Knitting is my hobby, and I find it invaluable to have a little corner of my life that's creative, enjoyable and entirely within my* control. If you don't have a hobby, think back to what you did when you were a child. Our young instincts for what we like – before we've learned what we ought to like – are pretty unerring. If you liked drawing, buy a sketch book and some good pencils and join a life-drawing class. If the school play was the highlight of your year, find a drama group nearby and throw yourself in.

- Bit-of-organizing things, like going out for a coffee with a friend, or going to the cinema, or arranging to go for a bike ride with someone, or meeting up with an old colleague during their lunchhour.

- Big things, like planning a holiday, or tracing your family history, or sorting out all of your photographs.

Once you have your list, decide how you are going to use it. Unless you have a magic notebook, a list is only as much use as what you do with it afterwards. So decide how you are going to use these ideas to fill the well: are you going to block out space in your diary, set aside a half-hour every day, take every other Saturday morning, or fit in well-filling as and when you can, and keep a note of it? It doesn't matter how you decide to fill your well, so long as you do it, and you do it enough for there to be something for you to take when you need to.

BLOG POST, 25 MAY 2011 (ABRIDGED): A RAINBOW

Monday in Scotland and the north east of England was stormy and windy. By the end of Monday, much of Scotland had power cuts and the gale force winds were wreaking havoc.

I was in Edinburgh and got on my train home at 6:30 p.m. feeling more than a little lucky. The departure board at the station had been a parade of 'cancelled', the concourse bursting with people wailing, 'I don't know what to do now, there's not a hotel room to be had in Edinburgh' into their phones. Yet my train left just 20 minutes after it said it was going to. (As I have been known to leave just 20 minutes after I said I was going to, I found this easy to forgive.)

The train line from Edinburgh to Alnmouth is a thing of beauty. The rails dance along by the sea, sometimes almost close enough to touch, sometimes further away, but always in sight of each other. As I looked out of the window, the fields were the brilliant green of the just-been-hammered-with-rain, the sea the colour of a fading bruise, the sky a dirty shade of Earl Grey tea.

And then I saw a rainbow. It was, to be fair, one of the worst rainbows I've ever seen. Faint and feeble, a little bit grubby, starting at the sea and barely getting into its curve before the cloud devoured it.

But a rainbow is a rainbow, and a rainbow does two things to me: it gives me a little hit of beauty and excitement, and it makes me want to show someone else. There was a little girl with her family sitting across the aisle from me. I looked over… she was asleep. I didn't think her parents would appreciate it if I woke her, especially as they were asleep too so I'd have to wake them to ask them if I could wake her.

So I didn't show anyone else the rainbow. And afterwards, I wished I had. There were other candidates: lots of benign-looking women reading books, a mildly flirtatious man in a suit… should I have mentioned it to one of them? Surely everyone wants to see a rainbow?

BAH! THINKING

Looking into the well

Get very still, and very quiet. Breathe in deeply, and out deeply, and breathe in more deeply, and breathe out more deeply, then in and out once again, more deeply still, and then allow your breathing to find a comfortable, quiet rhythm.

Take that forest path again. Walk slowly and feel the earth give beneath your feet. Feel comfortable. When you have walked far enough, you will come across a well. This is your well. It might be a fairy-tale well, built out of stone with a slanting tiled roof and a tin bucket. It might be little more than a hole in the ground with a tripod of sticks over the top. Maybe there's a handle to turn, maybe you pull on a rope to get the water. It's your well; you decide.

Sit down next to your well. Feel how comfortable you are. Feel how right this place seems to be: how nurturing, how easy. Feel how glad you are to be here, and how relaxed you have become as you sit here.

When you are ready, take a look into the well. See how full it is. Throw in a pebble and count if you want to find out how deep it is. Feel happy that you have this well, and that it's ready for you when you need it.

When you are ready, open your eyes.

Whenever you do something that is filling the well, remember how good it feels to be there and what a good thing you are doing for yourself.

Whenever you take something from the well, remember how much there is to draw from.

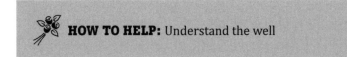

HOW TO HELP: Understand the well

At this point with your loved one, you will have understood – perhaps thanks to painful circumstances and difficult times – that you are only responsible for your own behaviour: that you cannot make the person in your life who is dancing with cancer do the things you think they ought to do. In other words, you cannot fill their well for them. But there are things that you can do.

- If you are both reading this book, use the language. Ask yourselves what you've done to fill the well lately. Say: 'I thought if we went out for lunch on Saturday it would fill the well a little more.'

- Fill your own well. You need resources to draw on just as much as your beloved does.

- Unobtrusively provide things that will help fill the well. Suggest a bath. Bring home a DVD. Arrange to see friends.

I've said this before, but I'm saying it again because it matters. The fact that you have survived cancer – and you are on your way to thriving afterwards – doesn't mean that you now have to enter – and win – every Mr/Ms Relentlessly Cheery 24/7 competition you come across. You are allowed to feel good. You are allowed to have a spring in your step, feel positive and be glad to be alive. You are entitled to nurture yourself and do everything you can to keep the well filled. But you are also allowed to feel lousy, tired, overwhelmed, fed up, resentful and so full of tears that they will spill over at the smallest drop of spilt milk. If you didn't feel that way sometimes, there would be something wrong. Let the bad days happen. Don't wallow; don't let them get out of control; reach into the well and find a way to take the edge off. And remember: part of being well is feeling a little bit lousy sometimes. It's OK. You're OK.

BAH! THINKING

The three-minute misery

Here's a strategy for when you are having One of Those Days.

Take a pen and a piece of paper.

Set a timer for three minutes, or take note of the time.

Spend these three minutes writing down everything that's annoying you, everything that's difficult, all that's unbearable right now. Write furiously (haha!), get your thoughts down and don't hold back.

At the end of the three minutes, take that piece of paper, tear it up into little pieces and throw it in the bin. Preferably a bin with a lid, so you can slam it afterwards.

Go about your day knowing that you've got rid of all that bad feeling.

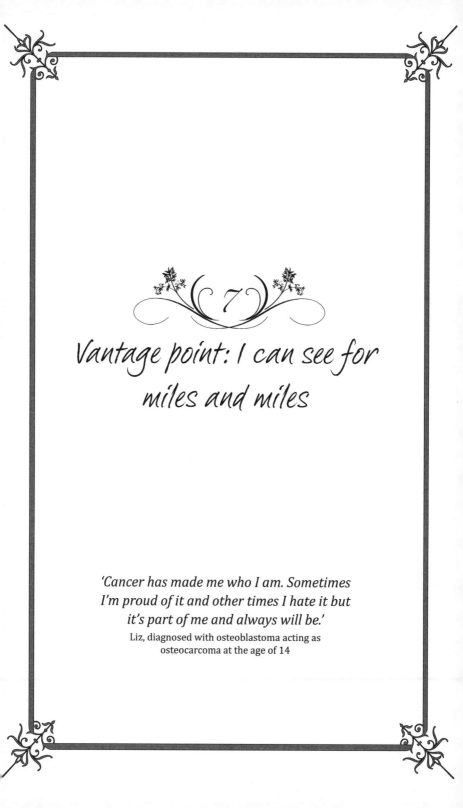

7

Vantage point: I can see for miles and miles

'Cancer has made me who I am. Sometimes I'm proud of it and other times I hate it but it's part of me and always will be.'

Liz, diagnosed with osteoblastoma acting as osteocarcoma at the age of 14

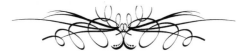

There are things that people say, when they are talking about cancer. You hear these things repeated over and over in radiotherapy waiting rooms, as chemotherapy snakes into veins, at wig-wearing workshops and queues at reception desks where we wait to make the next appointment. We say them to the friends who are with us as we wait to see our consultants; we say them on the phone as we call to cancel an appointment or shift a meeting because we aren't well, or because cancer is surreptitiously munching through our diaries as though the days of our lives are about as significant as the sugar on a doughnut.

I used to think of these things as cancer clichés, because everyone said them, all the time, and they became meaningless. I tried to avoid saying them myself, fearing being obvious, or boring, or thoughtless. But then I realized that the reason we all say these things, all of the time, is not because the words are easy or mindless or dull: it's because the words are true.

Somewhere on the road to thriving, there's a fresh outlook born of an accumulation of the whole cancer experience: every phone call, every needle, every long afternoon, get-well-soon card, sleepless night and left-field side-effect combined and processed somewhere between the heart and brain and the place where your soul resides.

I had a conversation with a lovely woman who had danced with cancer more than 20 years ago. (I LOVE meeting people like that.) 'The thing is,' she said sheepishly, 'all I really learned from cancer was that life is short and not worth wasting. It's hardly earth-shattering.' Maybe not. But it doesn't matter. First, because learning something for yourself is infinitely more valuable than being told it. Of course, even without a cancer we know that life is short. But we don't feel it until we've been in rooms with people using words like 'prognosis' and 'tumour' and 'lymph nodes'. (Just like listening to someone telling you how good their pecan pie tastes isn't the same as eating it yourself.) And the second reason it doesn't matter how earth-shattering your insight is, is that it's the impact it has that matters. The woman I was talking to had taken what she thought of as her run-of-the-mill new perspective and turned it into two decades of fresh experiences and enthusiasm. I could see the value of the perspective cancer had given her, shining out of her face as she talked.

That's when I stopped thinking about cancer clichés, and embraced cancer insights. Here they are. I know that you'll recognize them. That's what's so brilliant about them.

CANCER MAKES YOU REALIZE WHAT'S IMPORTANT IN YOUR LIFE

I'm much better at cherishing my family, my friends, my health and my home now. There are other things that have turned out to be important, too. Beaches – big, empty or nearly-empty beaches, sand studded with hoofprints, pawprints, footprints and initials drawn with sticks, water any shade of monochrome or blue. Beaches matter. (I'm one of several people thriving after cancer I know of who have moved to be near the sea. I wonder if, on some level, our bodies choose or need the air, the salt, the sky big enough to fit the whole of a rainbow in.) Making things with my hands, and giving them to people that matter to me, with love knitted or sewn or mixed into every stitch or bite. Helping: picking through my dance with cancer and finding ways to use what I learned to help others. These things matter, and a lot of others don't. Within two weeks of diagnosis I'd ditched my psychology degree, because I could see that I wasn't really getting what I'd hoped for from it. Similarly, my cake business went within three months, partly because I was afraid of letting people (especially brides) down, and partly because my fresh eyes showed me that I didn't enjoy the business half as much as I thought I was going to when I began it. I'm fairly confident that, without cancer, I would still be spending every Saturday from May to September driving a five-tier confection around the country and weeping at every speed bump while fretting about the Open University coursework as yet undone. Don't get me wrong, I wasn't actively unhappy before – well, maybe at some of the more disastrous speed-bumpy parts – I was just too busy to take a look at the calibre of the life I was leading or, more often than not, being led by.

CANCER MEANS YOU FIND OUT WHO'S TRULY IN YOUR CORNER

And some of those people surprised me. Distant colleagues started to send me daily emails telling me how well I was doing, and that it would all be just fine. I got cards, flowers, gifts, you-can-do-it texts from corners of my life that I wouldn't have expected. Conversely, a couple of friends I'd known for years sent me 'so sorry to hear that' emails and promptly vanished for a year, presumably to minimize their chances of catching a cancer themselves. Others didn't quite seem to grasp that when I said I couldn't do something, I truly couldn't do it, I wasn't just feeling sorry for myself. (Not that I never felt sorry for myself. I was just good at recognizing and admitting it when I was.)

YOU ARE STRONG; YOU CAN DO IT

OK, you don't have a choice. Well, you do: you can sign the consent forms, have the surgery, suck up the chemotherapy and the side-effects, live a life you would never have chosen and hope that it will end with some sort of happy – or you can lie down and die. And the funny thing is, before I was diagnosed I would have sworn blind that I would have chosen that second option, written pretty goodbye-and-thank-you notes and popped a bedjacket on ready for when the gentleman with the scythe came for me. Not that I wanted to die: no, I was 100% convinced that I simply didn't have whatever I imagined it took to endure a dance with cancer. Every now and then I'd see a fellow patient looking bemused as they smiled at the nurse plugging in another drip of something nasty, and I'd think they, too, are thinking, 'Well, look at me, who'd have thought I could do this?' I don't know whether I'm stronger than I thought I was, or whether the physical instinct for survival overrides the brain's constructions of ourselves as unable to withstand something like cancer. Maybe it's a bit of both. I don't think that matters. What matters is that now we know we can do it.

EVERYTHING PASSES

The good and the bad.

LIFE GOES ON

Your life. Everyone else's life. And the life around you, even if it happens without you. Cancer made me feel like a very teeny tiny speck of universe indeed. And I'm glad of that, because I think that insight freed me from the pre-cancer way I lived, when everything mattered so terribly, terribly much, and I was anxious and competitive as a result.

I'm not sure that these Standard Cancer Insights are much to do with cancer, really. I think they are to do with having a short, sharp shock of mortality combined with a lot of thinking time. (Listen to someone who's had a dance with cancer and someone who's had a bereavement and you'll find a great deal of overlap.) Not that it matters. The fact is, cancer is likely to give you a new perspective on your life.

BAH! THINKING

What's your perspective?

It's time to revisit the notebook and the quiet place.

Take a double-page spread. One side is going to be for the good things that have happened as a result of cancer. The other is for the things that you might not be comfortable with.

On the top of the left-hand page, write 'I know/believe...'

Underneath it, list everything that you've learned, or seen afresh, during your dance with cancer. It doesn't matter if it's obvious. It doesn't matter if it's trivial, or embarrassing. No one is going to see it, unless you invite them to. So what if you now love your hair as much as you love your children? So what if it's taken you this much of your life to work out that your dad is, despite his faults, still a pretty good father?

What you've done, in effect, on that first page, is create your own personal manifesto for living. It might not be something that you need – you're unlikely to be asked to produce it at a job interview, and, although it's a long time since I've been on the dating scene, I don't remember it being high on the list of first-date questions – but it's something that's reassuring to have. I think of mine as an anchoring point in my life.

And how fantastic is it to go through life really, truly knowing what you are about, and understanding what's important to you, and feeling that knowledge and understanding play out through your days, your relationships, your decisions?

Pretty fantastic.

Now turn to the facing page. On the top, write 'I wonder...'

This is the place for the things you wonder about, you're not sure of, or you feel are unresolved. Without overthinking, write down the things in your life now that you aren't happy about, or you have yet to make peace with. Perhaps you don't know how you feel about dying. Perhaps you are angry that a friend let you down. Maybe you can't seem to come to terms with the way your body – or you – behaved during treatment. Whatever it is, put it on the page.

Now turn to a fresh page. Take a look at each item on each list, and write down what actions you need to take to move things on, if any. You're more likely to need to take action on the 'wonder' list, because there may be things there that are unresolved.

Some of the things on your 'wonder' list will require practical effort. You might feel that you need to apologize to someone, or tell them how you feel. If you're unhappy with your treatment you may need to write a letter to the place where you were treated and ask for an explanation or an investigation. Make a note of what you will do, and when you will do it by.

There will be other things on your 'wonder' list that you can't take practical action on, but which you need to let go of. We're coming to that next.

Before we do: a final word on the manifesto you have just created. Nothing on it is written in stone, and so it's probably worth an annual review. After all, our vantage point changes as we make any journey.

BAH! THINKING

A visualization for letting go

Find somewhere quiet and calm where you will be undisturbed. When you are ready, close your eyes and breathe deeply until your mind is still and your breath comes and goes evenly and without effort.

Imagine yourself on a hillside, high and bright under the happy sky of your choosing. The air is clear, you are comfortable and relaxed and happy. There is no one nearby and the view in front of you is still and peaceful, with a clear view to the sea on the horizon.

Imagine taking a balloon from your pocket. Now, deliberately bring to mind something that you are struggling to let go of. Hold that thing in your mind, and when your mind is full of it, bring the balloon to your lips and blow that thing into it. (This is a visualization, so the balloon inflates without that tricky first stage where you have to make a gargantuan effort to get the rubber to start stretching and you can feel blood vessels bursting in your eyeballs.) Blow up the balloon, fuller and fuller, until it is full of the thing you are letting go of and your head is empty of it. When the balloon is full, tie off the end and let it go. Watch it as it floats off towards the sea. Keep on watching it – don't take your eyes from it – until it vanishes over the horizon. Feel the relief as the balloon vanishes. Enjoy that moment.

When the balloon has gone, take another from your pocket. Fill your mind with another thing that you need to let go of, and blow it into the balloon like you did before. When your mind is empty, tie up the balloon, let it go and watch it until it has disappeared, too.

Keep on pulling balloons out of your pocket until your mind is free of everything you need to let go of.

When the last balloon has gone, spend a minute or two feeling how good it is to be free of those lingering thoughts. Remind yourself that they really have gone. They have. You just saw them disappear, with your own eyes.

When you are ready, take some deep, slow breaths, smile the smile of the freshly unburdened, and open your eyes.

I worked with someone who was so taken with the idea of this visualization she decided to go a step further by blowing up balloons and releasing them in her garden, watching them float away. She chose a windy day so it worked well, until a balloon snagged and burst on the top of a tree in her garden. She had to spend all winter watching a piece of stranded orange rubber, and couldn't let go of the thought it symbolized until it was eventually dislodged by a spring gale…

If you want to take this visualization and make it into a physical exercise, you could write each thought onto a piece of paper, wrap it tightly round a pebble and throw it into the sea, over a waterfall or into the fast-moving, endless form of water of your choice.

BLOG POST, 10 DECEMBER 2010 (ABRIDGED): UNDERSTANDING

There are people I would, I think, have imagined I'd get much more help and care from, and others who surprised me in what dedicated and thoughtful friends they turned out to be.

To start with, I subscribed to the conventional view: cancer (like any other life crisis where you are likely to need to lean on people) means that you find out who your friends are. But I've come to realize that it's not that simple.

I think that the support we can offer each other depends on how much we have going on at the time ourselves: we have finite resources, physical and emotional, and the help we can give to others comes from the surplus from our own lives. But we don't always see that. I remember when a dear and close friend of mine got divorced. She wasn't happy about it – it wasn't her idea – and, as she lived too far away to visit, I resolved that I would call her once a week, every week, to see how she was doing. And I did. For the first two weeks. And then... well, I was up to my ears in small children and a new job and other things, and, somehow, it was Christmas before I picked up the phone again. I really wasn't the friend I wanted to be, and I'm ashamed that I didn't do more. And I'm sure that's not the only time someone else's life crisis has passed me by because I didn't have the resources right then to help.

So I've tried to understand all the people I know who've been busy wiping little noses or being bereaved or feeling that they need to focus on their own hopes and needs right now. I've tried to keep at the forefront of my mind that, although someone not being there when you need them can feel like the most direct and intimate of rejections, it's not really personal. And I've tried to keep my end of things up too. I haven't always had a lot of resources myself, but I've tried to keep on being the best mother and wife and friend that I can be. I haven't always done it very well, and I know that, and the people in my life know that, too. But most of us understand, I think, that we are doing what we can. And that act of understanding makes life easier.

Cancer, after all, is just another bit of stuff that can happen in life. Births, deaths, marriages, new babies, divorces, new jobs, redundancies, love in the shape of someone you'd never have thought of, house moves, strokes of good fortune, illnesses sudden and creeping – they all go on, all the time, for all of us. Those of us dancing with cancer need to remember this, even when having a cancer feels like lying on the slow lane of the M1 while the juggernauts keep coming. Others will do what they can for us – and though that 'what they can' may be great or small, we need to appreciate that and try to do the same in our turn.

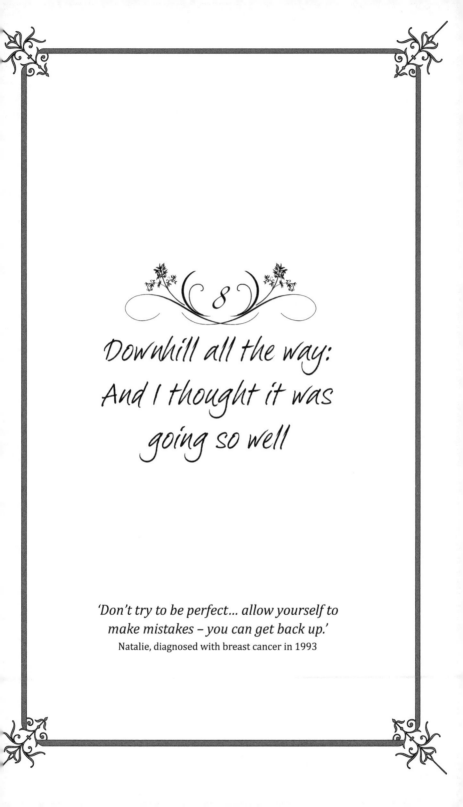

8

Downhill all the way: And I thought it was going so well

'Don't try to be perfect... allow yourself to make mistakes – you can get back up.'
Natalie, diagnosed with breast cancer in 1993

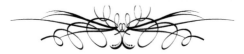

Shortly after I was diagnosed with breast cancer, I sent an email to a woman I knew only slightly: she was organizing an event I had said I would go to, but as it was going to be the week after surgery I was sending my apologies instead. I got a swift and matter-of-fact reply: 'Of course. I understand – I've had breast cancer too, four years ago now. Don't worry. You'll be fine.' I smiled and put this message in the part of my mind directly opposite the place where all of the 'Oh no! You poor, poor thing! My auntie died of breast cancer!' messages were stored. (It was early days. I hadn't yet learned that I didn't have to store those second sort of messages at all.)

About 15 minutes later I had another message from the same woman. 'I should have said – be warned,' it read, 'the worst time can actually be about six months after you finish treatment, when what you've been through suddenly hits you, and you can hit a real low. It happened to me and several others I know who've had cancer. Make sure you keep taking care of yourself.'

I'd been depressed, on and off, for the best part of a decade, so this advice struck me as being really important, and I held on to it. As it happened, I managed to circumvent this particular pit – I think it's a lot to do with my almost-daily blogging, which allowed me to process my experience in little, manageable chunks – but I've seen and heard about it from others. I don't think it's an experience common to cancer – I think any time in our lives which either demands extraordinary strength or causes intense pressure has to have an after-effect. (I cried for two days after seeing Duran Duran in concert in my teens. That's still pretty much how I work.)

BAH! THINKING

Plan for the dark times

This might seem counterintuitive, especially coming from me with my (undeserved) reputation for relentless cheerfulness. But, as I've said on many occasions when I've been asked how I manage to be so positive all the time, as though I'm some sort of deranged, grinning mannequin made flesh: being positive is not about pretending to be happy if you're not. It's about recognizing when positive action is needed, and taking it.

When you are already feeling low is not the time to start trying to look after your mental health, in the same way that standing on the starting line of a marathon is not the time to start thinking about training for it. (There's only so far expensive trainers and Deep Heat will take you, and it ain't 26 miles.) So here are some strategies for making sure you're prepared.

- *Look ahead. Are there times when you know there's a good possibility that you might need a bit of emotional support? These times might be cancer anniversaries – diagnosis, surgery, a tough time with treatment or, conversely, the date when treatment stopped and you found yourself standing on the steps of the hospital, drifting, with the appointments, treatments and meetings that had moored you gone. They might be non-related anniversaries – a parent's death, the date of your first disastrous marriage that you can't forget because you looked forward to it for so very long. Or it could be that the few days after the clocks change disorient you, the dark days at the end of February bring you down... it could be anything. What it is isn't important. What's important is that you see it coming and act accordingly. Arrange to go for a walk, see a film, go out for dinner, be away on a course.*

- *Ask for help. Take those dates and ask your loved ones to mark the date in their diaries. If the day comes and you feel fine, then that's great: you still get to do the well-filling thing, you still get a bit of extra love and attention from the people who care for you. If the day comes and you don't feel fine, you have something to tide you over.*

- *If moods and down times don't seem to have any rhyme or reason, check. In a diary, rate your days and see if you can see a pattern – are there places you go, people you see, jobs that you do that might be triggering a reaction in you? Is there a correlation with coffee, or alcohol, or sleep, or how many hours you spend working on your* computer or what time you switched off the TV the night before? This sounds like hard work – but I think having dark days is harder. Especially if you can get rid of them with a fairly minor lifestyle change. I find that having hot water with a squirt of lemon juice first thing in the morning is profoundly cheering – no matter how much tea and coffee I drink later. I've no idea why it works, but it does, so I do it.

- Practise acceptance. If I'm not feeling 100% chirpy, I can get into a tailspin of panic and misery. I forget that, sometimes, it's possible to be in a bad mood or have an off day because, actually, that's just normal. It doesn't mean the beginning of depression: that sound I hear isn't the clanging chimes of doom. If you don't feel fantastic, note that to yourself and get on with what you were doing. If you find it hard to do this, write it down somewhere. I write 'This too shall pass' on bits of paper and put them in places where I'll see them often: the noticeboard above my desk, folded into my purse, as a bookmark in whatever I'm reading.

- Know the signs. I used to find that by the time I noticed I was down and said something, my family would respond with, 'You haven't been quite yourself for the last couple of days.' So now, when I feel as though someone is asking me if I'm OK with infuriating frequency, rather than getting annoyed with them I realize that I'm probably not quite OK.

- Get into the habit of talking about how you feel. On good days, tell your loved ones that you feel great/excited/

happy. When you have a big occasion coming up, discuss feeling nervous and excited. If the only time you ever really talk about feelings is when you're low, it will be all the more difficult. Set a precedent in your relationships for talking about how you are, however you are.

Unfortunately, it's in the nature of depression that you don't recognize it until it's too late. You're not depressed: you've simply noticed how bloody awful life is, and all of these people around you being cheerful and enjoying life are just deluded. But there are things you can do – steps you can take, both physical and mental – that might keep the shadows at bay. Depression is terrible, but it's not compulsory.

BAH! THINKING

The good in everything

Take a notebook. Maybe not your usual notebook: maybe another one, small enough to slip into a pocket or your handbag. And when I say take it, I mean take it everywhere. And every time you see something that makes you smile, or something good happens to you, make a note in that book. It might be just a word or two – 'great coffee', 'seat on the train', 'sex'. (I chose those at random, by the way, I'm not designing my dream morning.) You might want to make a tick or a tally mark, rather than actually record the details of the good thing. Or you might hold on to the thought until you reach a place where you can describe it more fully. Experiment and find a way that works for you. (It might not even be a notebook. It might be something you set up on your phone. The crucial thing is that you have something to hand all the time to record good things. And they don't have to be major good things: this is not a place only for marriage proposals, pay rises, new babies and reaching remission dates. Though I would hope those things would make it onto your list.)

What's important here is that you are actively noticing good things around you, and recording them. This will help you to create a frame of mind in which you begin automatically noticing things that make you happy, rather than things that bring you down.

And your record will give you something to go back to when you feel as though life is unrelentingly awful.

As time goes on you might find that noticing good things has become part of your daily habit, and so you no longer feel the need to write them down. That's fine, so long as you're aware if the habit starts to slip, and then you take up your notebook and pen again.

You might want to tell the people close to you about some of your good things, whether it's hitting every green light on the journey home or the rain stopping just as you stepped out of the door. A joy shared is a joy multiplied. (Or something.)

BLOG POST, 9 JUNE 2010 (ABRIDGED): A PEARL

A few weeks ago, I was at my yoga class, creaking and cramping my way valiantly through. I was getting a bit disheartened, and thinking how glad the rest of the class must have been when I joined because I was living proof that they were better at yoga than (a) they thought (b) me. (Yes, yes, we all know that yoga is about what your body can do today and it's not competitive… but I'm sure it takes at least 20 years of practice before you mean that, rather than just say it.)

So. I was struggling. There are things that my body just can't do at the moment: my spine is more or less locked solid from shoulder blades to waist; my hamstrings are getting stronger but still aren't what they could (will) be; my arms are weak, especially the post-PICC left one.

One transition in particular, though, everyone was finding tricky. Our teacher, Lisa, watched us for a while, thudding and galumphing on our mats as we more-or-less managed the physical actions, but in a way that would make even the most zen of teachers weep. She stopped us, and demonstrated, talking us slowly through each movement as she did it, explaining what was happening in her joints and muscles. At one point we needed to make space to move one foot to between our hands. 'If you are struggling,' said Lisa, 'lift up your heart.'

Of course, what she was trying to get us to do was to widen our shoulders, stretch our necks, keep our spines long. As a physical instruction, it worked well.

But for me, this instruction worked, in a much bigger way. (It's not the first time yoga has had an

107

emotional as well as a physical effect.) During a break in a difficult meeting a couple of weeks later, I said to myself, 'When you are struggling, lift up your heart.' I walked back in straighter and stronger. When I'm tired or not feeling up to much, I remember my teacher's words and I think of my heart, think of it lifting, and I find it impossible not to take a deep breath and smile. (I'm writing this on a train and I did it just now. I'm grinning like an idiot.)

So. Another example of the power of words. I offer this phrase to you and invite you to take it and use it if it speaks to you, too.

When you are struggling, lift up your heart.

BAH! THINKING

A meditation for how you feel today

Get still. Get quiet.

Close your eyes and take three deep breaths in and out, then let your breathing settle into a peaceful, easeful rhythm.

Quietly ask yourself the question: 'How do I feel today?'

Don't rush to answer the question. Wait. Breathe. See what happens.

Something will come to you, like a bubble rising to the top of a pond. It might be a word, a feeling or an image.

Take a good look at it. Treat it the way you'd treat a waking animal: give it lots of space, don't make any sudden movements, let it be.

The feeling might have surprised you, or it might be familiar. It doesn't matter. What's important is to take a moment, now, to accept the feeling. Even if you feel angry or upset or sad, and you know that you'll want to take steps to feel better – the first step to that is to embrace the feeling. Welcome it. Tell it that it's just fine as it is.

When you are ready, open your eyes, take a deep breath and do whatever you need to do – perhaps you want to hold on to the feeling, perhaps you want to move on and feel differently. Either is easier once you have accepted what the starting point is.

Feeling low is an understandable and necessary part of the journey from surviving a dance with cancer to thriving after it. We wouldn't be human – or honest – if we claimed that life after cancer was an unending parade of ecstasy and delight. Depression, however, is a serious illness in its own right.

If your occasional down days turn into weeks, if you feel incapable of feeling, if you can comfortably describe your life as a prison or a hole or bleak, or you genuinely wish you were dead, you need to get help. At the very least, the help of talking to someone else, preferably a professional. Depression is a disease in the same way that cancer is a disease, and needs to be treated as such. If you broke your leg, you wouldn't walk on it, and depression is another way that the body can be broken. Don't suffer. Or rather, if you are suffering, take steps to make the suffering stop, however pointless those steps might appear right now.

And keep drawing from your well. That's what it's there for.

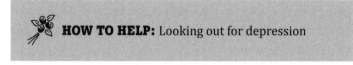

HOW TO HELP: Looking out for depression

If your beloved seems low, or starts to behave differently, you may need to take action. Classic symptoms of depression can include, but aren't limited to: lethargy, sleeplessness, crying, not wanting to do very much, loss of appetite and sex drive, loss of interest in things that the person is usually passionately interested in, neglected appearance. Someone who is depressed isn't always open to the idea of getting help – because it seems pointless – so it can be a difficult thing to manage. Here are some suggestions.

- Monitor their moods/behaviour so that when you have a conversation with them you can give clear examples of when they haven't seemed like themselves. (This isn't a list of their failings: it's more, 'You cancelled your trip to the cinema, but you didn't seem to have any reason why, and I know it was a film you really wanted to see.')

- Talk about how you feel, not what they might be feeling. If you start to speculate on what someone else is feeling, it's easy to upset them and/or to get it wrong, and that's the end of the conversation, right there. If you say, 'When I look at you I see someone who appears tired and unhappy and not themselves, and that makes me unhappy, and it makes me want to help,' you make it much easier for your loved one to respond.

- If there seem to be regular points in the day or week when your loved one struggles, try – unobtrusively – to arrange things to occupy them during that time. This won't help to overcome a serious depression, but it might help to make for fewer bad days.

- Don't try to counter misery with relentless cheerfulness. Be genuine and authentic.

- If you are really concerned, don't be put off. Keep talking, keep asking, keep suggesting a visit to the GP. Depression tends to take the line of least resistance, so if your loved one knows that you aren't going to give up, they will go along with you. ('Owt for peace', as we say in the north.)

- Read about depression yourself. It's one of those things – a bit like cancer – that we all think we understand but, when faced with it, we discover that we have a lot of preconceptions and assumptions about it. The more you know, the better you will cope. There are recommendations in the Resources chapter.

- Remember that the depressed person can't help the way they are behaving. They aren't wilfully looking for difficulties. And remember that they will come through depression. Remind them that they will.

- Don't stop planning. Trying to make plans with someone who is depressed can turn into a mighty long session of, 'Why don't we...?' 'I can't, because...' Don't be put off. Keeping someone who is depressed in the world is one of the best things you can do for them.

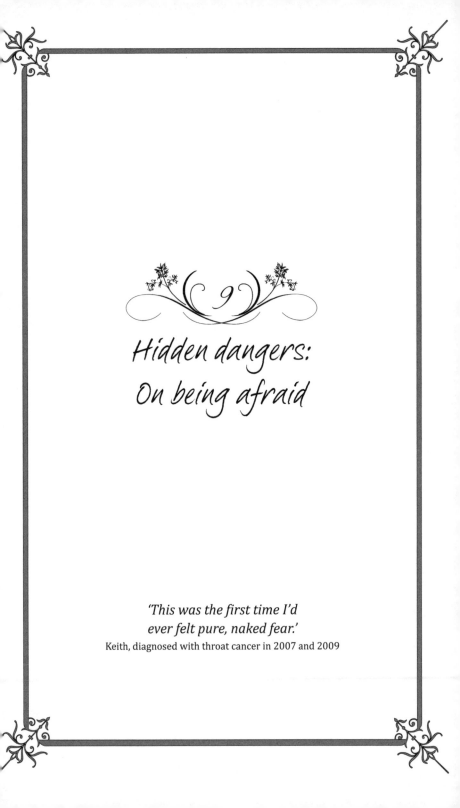

9

Hidden dangers:
On being afraid

*'This was the first time I'd
ever felt pure, naked fear.'*
Keith, diagnosed with throat cancer in 2007 and 2009

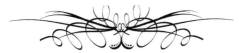

People often tell me that I'm brave, and I smile and say, 'Thank you.'

It's taken me a while to get to the realization that smiling and saying 'Thank you' is the only response to this. I used to say that, actually, if that person had a cancer they would be just as brave, if not braver, than me, because I'm pretty wimpy, really, especially when it comes to pointy things that hurt or the merest suggestion that medication might make me sick. I thought this was an encouraging thing to say, but the looks on people's faces when I said 'if you had a cancer' told me that offering them even this most hypothetical of cancers was not a good thing to do. So then I would try to suggest that, although they might not have had a cancer, they had probably been just as brave in a different way, or a different situation. That conversation sometimes went well, but more often degenerated into polite desperation, with each of us trying to find reasons why the other was the bravest. It was the diametric opposite of two new grandmas showing off their babies to each other, each believing that their own grandchild is the most beautiful baby that has ever existed.

So. When someone tells me I am brave, I smile and I say, 'Thank you.'

And I suppose I *am* brave in the sense that, when it came to it, I submitted to some grim stuff and stood up for myself when I needed to. I give talks, during which I stand in front of a projected image of my scarred breasts. I blog about how it feels to be thriving after cancer on days when I'd much prefer to quietly pretend that it never happened.

But I do think bravery is overrated, and brave faces can be counterproductive. Fear is a completely reasonable reaction to cancer, and to the prospect of cancer returning.

BLOG POST, 21 JANUARY 2012 (ABRIDGED): AFRAID

This week I was on the radio. The other guest and I were both asked what we were afraid of.

The other guest's impressively terrifying answer was 'being buried alive' – something I'm now scared of, too, although I'd never much thought about it before. My answer didn't need a moment's thought: I'm most afraid, I said, of getting a cancer again, or of someone I love getting a cancer.

Maybe that's the answer that you'd expect from me, but I surprised myself.

First because I'm not the type of person who would go up a ladder that would take me more than 5 feet off the ground. I'd never bungee jump or eat fire or ride bareback, and I cannot for the life of me understand why anyone would take part in any sport where falling off/over is part of the deal. (No cycling, skiing, skating for me.) So there are plenty of things that I'm properly scared of which are more immediately terrifying than cancer.

Then there's the fact that I know how cancer works and what it does. If I had a cancer again I'd be starting from an advantage: I'd be able to skip the whole finding-out, not-quite-knowing, why-me?, how-did-this-happen-to-me? disorienting bit at the beginning and go straight on to getting on with dancing it the hell out of my life, again.

Also, I know that I'd get through it. I know how many people I have to support me and love me well again. I know that there would be plenty of needles and nasty medicines with my name on them, all set to get the cancer gone. And I know I look marvellous in a hat, darling.

Although, maybe these reasons to *not* be scared of cancer are also the reasons that I *am*. Putting the people I love through a horrible time. Knowing exactly what I'd be in for. (Or having a fair idea, anyway.

117

I'm guessing every dance with cancer is different.) Knowing that there'd be the march of days where everything aches, and everywhere you go there's someone waiting with the latex gloves and the big, fat file of notes that document every drop of blood, every drip of drug, every trace of your heart. And that wellness would return, but that it would be a long time coming, and that I'd have to start being patient all over again.

There are many things that I could make myself afraid of if I thought about them. But I suppose I never have to, and choose not to: I don't believe that wondering in advance about something terrible happening to my family would make me any better equipped should the time come. Cancer, I do think about. Cancer, I am afraid of.

Although, funnily enough, I feel a lot better for saying so.

BAH! THINKING

What are you scared of?

Take a clean sheet in the notebook and a deep breath, and name your fears about cancer.

Obviously, cancer in itself is worth being scared of, but try to break it down into the bits that you are really frightened of. For example, my list reads:

- *horrible chemotherapy that I can't cope with*

- *needles*

- *pain*

- *my family being upset*

- *not being able to do what I want to do*

- *dying before I'm ready to*

- *dying a long drawn-out death*

- *letting people down. (Nobody says fears need to be rational.)*

Once you've done this, take another deep breath and feel proud of yourself for making your list. Fear exists for a reason: it's the brain's way of identifying dangers and making sure we stay safe. (Just think of what life would be like if your brain didn't warn you about traffic, food that smells funny or charming men who want to take your number but can't, at this moment, quite remember their own.) And a great deal of fear is learned behaviour. So, once we've danced with cancer our brains know that it's a completely reasonable thing to be frightened of. You know how you've never liked cats since the family pet bit your hand when you were six and you had to have a tetanus jab and stitches? It's that.

So when I open an envelope that contains an appointment for my annual better-safe-than-sorry mammogram, or the yearly come-in-for-a-chat-and-a-check-up with oncology, I'm frightened. I don't gibber or scream or take to my bed, but I do feel fear nipping gently at the edges of my heart. It's taken me a long time to realize that it's natural for this to happen, and that fear isn't a lapse or a sign of weakness. It's natural. But it does need to be kept in its place.

BAH! THINKING

A visualization for facing your fears

Get still and quiet.

Breathe, breathe deeply, breathe more deeply still.

When you are calm, walk back into your woods again. For myself, I visualize going through a gate to get to my woods, and so every time I close my eyes and imagine the gate, I immediately feel relaxed. But that's just my woodland. Yours is yours.

See how beautiful your wood is. It's bright and alive. It's green. It's safe.

Walk until you find a cluster of objects in a clearing.

This is the place where your fears are. These are your fears.

They might be in the form of people, or objects, or paintings, or sculptures. Your fears might simply be a list. It doesn't matter.

Take a deep breath, feel calm and walk towards the objects.

Look at each fear in turn. Really look at it. Don't let the fear sidle up to the corner of your eye then slide away from you again. Take each of your fears, one by one – pick them up if you want to – and examine them. Turn them over in your hands. If you fear a needle, take a good look at it, shining in the light. Run your finger down it. Test the tip of the needle against the tip of your finger.

As you hold and examine each object that you are afraid of, feel that you are seeing it as it really is. As you do so, let the fear in you drain away. Feel it pass down through your body, out of the soles of your feet into the earth. A needle becomes just a needle.

When you are ready, turn away from the place where your fears are. Feel how empty your body is, now that the fear has gone from it. And, as you stand in the bright, clean forest, feel something else fill the space where the fear was. Be filled with confidence that you can cope with the difficulties around you. Be filled with the knowledge of the strength that you have found. Be filled with light.

When you are ready, open your eyes.

Do this as often as you need to.

BAH! THINKING 🐉

An alternative to a visualization for facing your fears

If visualization is difficult for you, or if a lot of your fears are attached to physical objects – needles, tablets, hospital clinics – use the same process but in the real world. Find a needle and hold it in your hand. Arrive at the clinic early so you can spend half an hour sitting in a screwed-down chair and letting the fear drain through you and into the shade-of-green-no-one-would-really-choose carpet. If you're scared of losing your hair again, take out a headscarf and put it on while you let the fear dissipate.

BAH! THINKING 🐉
Practical strategies for when you are afraid

I'm a great believer in visualizations and the power of the mind. But there are times when you need a practical strategy too. Here are some ideas.

If something that you fear is causing you to lose sleep, lose weight, gain weight, or have panic attacks, or stopping you from being able to concentrate, work or function in your family, recognize that this is something you need help with. Talk to your GP or someone you trust from your time with hospital treatment. Don't wait to see if it improves. It won't, on its own.

Keep a diary of moods and fears. Write down when you feel fearful, where you are, what you were doing/about to do. Look for patterns. There might be one you haven't spotted, like being more afraid when a member of your family is away from home. (Remember, fear isn't linear.) And even if there is no pattern, having more information about when you feel fearful will help the people who are trying to help you.

When you're feeling afraid, try to think about what is behind your fears, as you did earlier in this chapter. People often tell me that they are now 'terrified of hospitals'. When I explore this some more, I usually find that it's not the hospital itself that they are afraid of. They are afraid of things that they associate with hospitals: pain, being ignored, being patronized, feeling ill, getting bad news. The more you can think about what, precisely, the fear is, the easier it is to deal with.

Remember, fears can change, or return, and that's natural. I don't think I'm afraid of needles anymore. I'm a lot more afraid of my family getting ill than I used to be. This makes sense to me: as my journey from survival to thriving goes on, I am less focused on my own pains/needs/world and a lot more aware of the people around me. So I need to be aware of these different fears, and be ready to take deep breaths and let my fears dissipate in new situations, while appreciating that it's a lot easier to have a blood test than it used to be.

Talk to the people around you. A brave face is not going to help you, or the people who want to support you.

This is a piece of completely partisan advice, because it's one of the best things I ever did: consider seeing a professional hypnotherapist.

Recognize that it is all right to be afraid. It's a normal response to a horrible thing. Cut yourself some slack. Say to yourself, 'Right now, I'm really scared of dying,' and allow that thought to sit with you. Sometimes, what causes problems for us isn't just fear but our attempts not to be afraid, which let the original feeling twist and grow into something much more complicated and difficult to deal with.

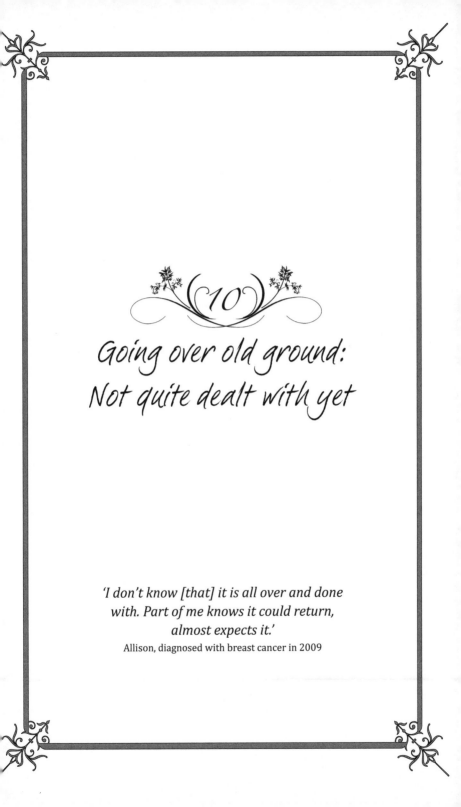

10

Going over old ground: Not quite dealt with yet

> 'I don't know [that] it is all over and done with. Part of me knows it could return, almost expects it.'
>
> Allison, diagnosed with breast cancer in 2009

Surviving cancer – well, surviving anything, really – is not a straight road. It can feel like taking three steps forward and two steps sideways sometimes. On really bad days, it's more like two steps sideways and then three back. It took me a long time to work out that, actually, that's OK. It's a natural part of the process to revisit, to go over again, to keep thinking about what has happened to you.

But I've found (I think) a better way to think of this than going backwards, however understandable and acceptable taking a few steps back is. Imagine – or take – a piece of A4 paper. Curl it into a cone. It will have a join running down inside it where the paper overlaps. The point at the bottom of the cone is the point where you begin to come to terms with something, and you make your way out by journeying in a spiral, round and round until you reach the top. The join is the thing that you are coming to terms with. So to begin with, you come across the difficulty on a really regular basis. You've barely sorted out your feelings when you hit it again. But as time goes on – as you start to progress up the spiral – you hit the difficulty less and less often. There's more smooth time and less bump. Eventually, the bump is only a tiny part of the continuing journey.

BAH! THINKING

A record of progress, and ghosts, and changes

Let's go back to the notebook.

Find a fresh page and write a list of the things that keep coming back to haunt you: the things you are going over again and again in your mind, or keep bumping up against in some other way.

When you've done that, give each thing on the list a score on a scale of 1 to 10. You are scoring how big a problem that thing is, right now, with 10 being 'This thing stops me from getting out of bed in the morning' and 1 is 'I'm aware of this but I really don't care about it at all.'

Take a look at anything scoring over a 7 or an 8 and ask yourself whether this is something that you need to take action on. That action might be as simple as explaining to someone else how you are feeling, or it may be that a conversation with your doctor is what's needed. It could be that you feel you want to note that this is hard right now, and wait. I have times when I feel overwhelmed by the memory of the frailty that came with cancer. I've found that the best thing to do is sit with that feeling, let it be part of me, and wait for it to go again. This, for me, has been more useful than talking about it, which makes the feeling more vivid, and more able to cling on.

For anything that scores 6 or under, just take a moment to acknowledge that this fear or flashback or memory is hanging around. Accept it as part of your life, for now. Resolve not to worry about it.

Every two weeks, come back to this list and score it again. Over time you'll see changes in how much old experiences are still having an impact on your life. If the trend is downward, you'll be able to see your progress, moving away from mere survival towards thriving. There may be the odd spike where fears become more important again, but that's all part of this rather uneven process.

My friend Nathalie has an interesting perspective on this part of the process of coming to terms with things. She told me about it one day shortly before we moved house, and I thought she was being ridiculous – but later she was proved right, and I felt a bit ridiculous myself.

I was explaining how rigorously I was packing. We were throwing out anything that was broken, missing any pieces or chipped. I refused to pack anything that had lain around unused for a few years, anything that we had a duplicate of, anything that had seemed like a good idea at the time. (The kitchen and the wardrobe were especially good places for those things to be hiding.) Everything from among these that wasn't broken went onto the front windowsill with a sign that said, 'Please help yourself.' Vases, odd wine glasses and travel-sized toiletries brought home from hotels far and wide were especially popular with people who were passing. I also got rid of the seven – yes, seven – bottles of soy sauce I'd somehow managed to accumulate. And someone took the chemotherapy headscarves I hadn't already sent on to other people in need of them. (I hoped that they weren't recognized as cancer paraphernalia, and would get a happy new life as napkins or dolly blankets.)

Nathalie listened to me patiently, and then said, well, yay me and all that, but when we came to unpack she guaranteed that I'd open boxes and have absolutely no idea why I'd packed the rubbish, tat and oddments that I found. 'You can only go so deep at any time,' she said. Yes, yes, I said, knowing in my heart that she was wrong because, although what she said might be true of other people, I was in fact a Ruthless Packing Ninja.

Then we moved into our new house, and took car-fulls of rubbish to the tip on a daily basis for what felt like months and months.

What Nathalie knew, and I had to learn, was this: at any point in time there's a limit to what you can let go of. There's only so much you can slough away in one attempt, whether we're talking emotions, cupboards-under-the-stairs or hard skin on your feet.

So it's not surprising that there are parts of our dance with cancer, and our journey to recovery, that we need to revisit. Before that conversation with Nathalie I often used to look back and wonder at some of the things that had happened to me, or that I had done. I wondered at the times when I thought I should have been physically stronger or mentally braver, or stood up for myself. But now I realize that, in those moments – when I was unwell, and almost certainly in pain, and probably tired and a little bit frightened – I was doing all that I could.

And I think that sometimes we need to keep revisiting old, difficult places until we can reconcile what we did then with what we would do now. So now, when I do find myself going back over something yet again, I reverse Nathalie's analogy and think of myself as adding another layer of compassion, of forgiveness, of understanding until one day, if I return to that place, I will do so without the feelings of distress that I've found there before.

BAH! THINKING 🐉

Revisiting

Think of somewhere that you love to walk, or cycle. It doesn't matter where it is, really, so long as you love it and can easily reach it. (For me, it's a local beach.)

Take your diary and put some time in it to take a walk/cycle in that place. Ideally, make appointments with yourself to go to that place six times over a two-week period. It doesn't have to be for long – a 20-minute walk will do – but commit yourself. Treat these walks/cycles as you would hospital appointments or best friends' birthday parties: you have to be there.

Then, come rain or shine, headache or bursting in-tray, take those six walks. Walk the same paths. Walk on your own, without music, without your phone. As you walk, breathe deeply. Feel your feet against the path, or earth, or sand, and let your eyes roam the landscape and pick out the details of the things you can reach out and touch.

If you want to, write down how you feel, what you saw, what happened, afterwards.

At the end of your six walks or rides, think back. Think about how different they were: about how, although you walked in the same place, each walk was different. The weather, the sky, the way your body felt as it moved, the day you were stepping away from, the things you turned over in your mind: all of the elements that gave you six separate experiences, each bringing you something new.

The next time you feel you are going round in circles, remember these walks. Go and take another one, if you feel like it. Remember that, although the place might be the same, you are not. See if you can bring something new away from your revisiting.

BLOG POST, 6 MAY 2010 (ABRIDGED): RELEASE

I want to tell you about a strange thing that happened at my yoga class this week. I'm not quite sure where to start, though. I guess I'll just plunge in and see what happens.

I'm gaining in strength and flexibility faster than I would have believed possible. However, bear in mind that my starting point was very weak and very stiff… so I am still fulfilling my role as the One at the Back of the Yoga Class that Everyone Is Reassured They Are Better Than, and will continue to do so for some time to come. Which is just fine by me.

At my class this week we did some standing postures that I haven't attempted since my return to yoga: some Trikonasana variations that require the legs to be stepped out and then the torso to twist, so there's a lot of movement in the spine. Now, right now, my spine is less a series of connected individual bones and more a broom handle, so anything that involves this kind of a twist is not easy. But the point of yoga is to do what you can, and breathe and release a little bit more into the posture, and a little bit more… until eventually you're so flexible that you can do the posture perfectly, and so serene that you don't care. (Allegedly.)

Anyway, everyone else in the class was getting a lot of a twist, and I was getting a bit of a twist, even if you would have needed a microscope to spot it, and congratulating myself on the fact that my legs could hold me up in this position, which they couldn't have done a month ago. And something released, and my spine twisted, maybe a millimetre more than it has done since my dance with cancer began.

And that's when the strange thing happened. With that millimetre of movement came the release of a wave of grief. It burst over me: a feeling of loss, of deep, true sadness.

I think that maybe the body stores memories of what affects it: that whatever happened to make that muscle knot – that moment of fear, or panic, or realization that cancer was actually here, actually inside me – got caught up with the muscle, somehow, so that when that knot of tension released, it let the emotion associated with it out, too. So I had a sort of time-capsule of tension, opened so that the grief that was captured poured out.

Of course I was not going to add to my 'worst-in-class' reputation by adding 'worst-in-class-and-bursts-into-tears-at-random-moments'. So I held on until I got home. And then I told Alan all about it and had a good cry. And then I felt better.

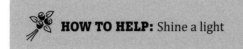

HOW TO HELP: Shine a light

Seeing someone you love start to thrive after cancer is a great thing, and it's easy to think that the best way to support them is to take the 'Don't Mention the War' approach, and keep all conversation very well clear of the c-word. But a dance with cancer is a trauma, and surviving it is a trauma – especially when we all know people who have died of cancer – and trauma grows into something ugly and unmanageable when it's kept in the dark. You can help your loved one to feel that it's OK to talk about the past.

- If something that happens in your everyday life reminds you of your loved one's dance with cancer, say so. It can be as simple as, 'When I went to buy lunch I saw someone with a scarf tied round their head and a shopping basket full of bananas and custard, and it reminded me of when you were having chemo and all you ate was rice pudding for a week.'

- Remember important dates. The day your loved one was diagnosed is likely to be right up there with birthdays and Christmas in their memory. Acknowledge these days when they come, quietly and kindly, so your loved one doesn't feel that everyone else has forgotten.

- When your loved one wants to talk about something related to cancer, always let them be the one to change the subject, or move the conversation on.

- Understand that your loved one may need to talk about the same thing over and over, as part of their coming to terms with it. Listen patiently, as often as it takes.

- Don't be afraid to talk about the things that upset or distress you. It's tempting to 'protect' your loved one from your feelings, but the more shared experience there is between you, the better for both of you. And your loved one will want to understand and help you in the same way that you do them; in fact, helping you may also help them to heal.

BAH! THINKING 🐉
Map-making

If you feel that you're going round in circles, and it's frustrating, then try this.

Take a big sheet of paper or a double-page spread in your notebook, and in the top right-hand corner write 'Thrive', or whatever word you associate with your ultimate wellbeing. If you're artily inclined, draw a symbol or picture for it, too. (For me, Thrive is a place of turrets and pennants and dragons perched on rooftops breathing benign and fragrant fire.)

The bottom left of the page is where you started. This is the place where you were when you first looked up and away from treatment, and thought, well, I've survived this after all.

Now make a map of your journey. The path you have followed may have been more downs than ups, or it might be a steady uphill trajectory. There's probably a roundabout somewhere, or a loop in the road. Stop drawing the path when you feel you've got to the point where you are today.

Now name some points on the map. 'Clear check-up' might be a high point, as might be the holiday you took to celebrate a year since diagnosis/surgery/last treatment. A jagged low might be the 'flu that felled you. That repeating circuit may be where you realized that, actually, getting better wasn't quite the five-minute job you were hoping for, and taking the last pill didn't mean that all of the pain and anxiety would vanish in the way you were half-hoping it would. The more detail you can add, the better.

When you have finished – for now, because you can go back to your map and add whatever you want to whenever you want to, until you get to the top right-hand corner – take a good look at your map. Maybe you'll want to run your finger along the pathway that you've drawn. Maybe you want to put your map on the wall, maybe you want to use it as a way to explain what you're going through. Perhaps the best thing for you to do is to turn the page and draw a new map next week. But whatever you decide to do with your map, before you do it take a moment to look at it and to understand how very far you have come. Acknowledge that some bits have been difficult. Look at the place where you went round in circles and think about what each circuit taught you. Remember just how deeply you breathed when you stood on those high points. And know that your path will keep on taking you in the right direction.

🌱 🌱 🌱

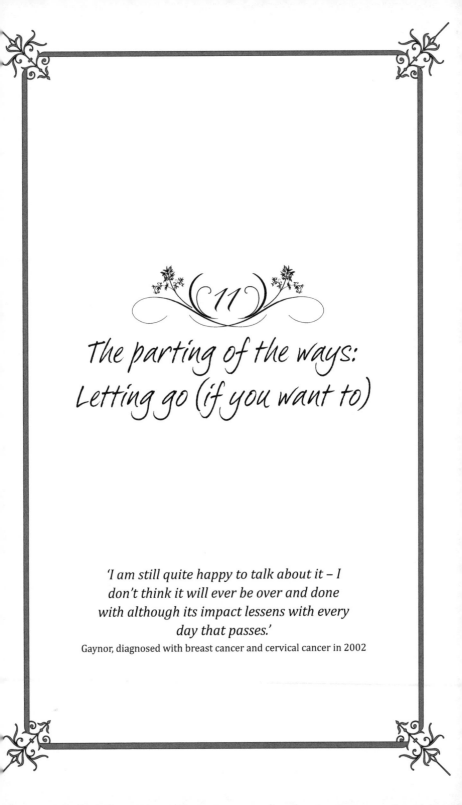

11

The parting of the ways:
Letting go (if you want to)

*'I am still quite happy to talk about it – I
don't think it will ever be over and done
with although its impact lessens with every
day that passes.'*

Gaynor, diagnosed with breast cancer and cervical cancer in 2002

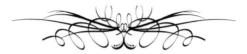

Cancer is a public disease. It's not discreet, and the symptoms and side-effects can't easily be explained away. So your chances of having cancer without a fairly wide circle of people knowing about it are slim.

But there comes a point in the journey to thriving when talking about cancer is no longer compulsory. You don't have to explain why you're not taking your hat off, even though you're indoors, because you have enough hair to be hatless – even if you do look as though you've made a very bold choice to go super-short. You can eat normal food at normal times. You don't jump and panic when someone sneezes within three feet of you.

At this point, you get a choice. You can be someone who leaves the cancer room via the door that goes back to where you were before you got the diagnosis, and get on with your life. Of course it won't be exactly the same, but near enough, and the benefit is that you never have to talk about cancer again if you don't want to, except to the people who you see once a year to reassure you that the tests say there's no sign of it coming back. After a while you may not even think about it that much anymore. As time rolls on, other people in your circle will have other crises, and yours will drift into history. This is the choice a lot of people make. They just want cancer to be over, and the more they talk about it, the less it is over. Therefore the less they talk about it, the happier they are. And that's fine.

BAH! THINKING 🦄

How to talk about cancer when you really don't want to talk about cancer

You may feel as though you never, ever want to mention the c-word again. But the likelihood is that it will come up now and again, so you might want to think about a way to say something about it, while making it clear that you aren't going to get into discussion.

Here are some suggestions. Use these as a starting-point, or take one and use it as it is. The important thing is that you feel confident with the words: that they are yours.

- *I had a cancer x years back. I'm fine now and I don't really talk about it anymore.*

- *Cancer is something that I went through. I'm so glad that I'm well now, and for me, part of wellness means that I try not to go back to that time.*

- *I had a cancer. I had surgery and chemotherapy and it took me about 18 months to get properly back on my feet. I really feel for people who are being diagnosed with cancer, but I don't feel that talking about my experience will help either them or me.*

- *I had a cancer. It wasn't a nice time in my life, but I did get through it and I think if you catch it early enough and look after yourself and take it one day at a time, then it's possible to get through fairly unscathed. I choose not to talk about it now because I'm looking to the future.*

Whatever you say, if you say it sincerely, most people will understand. Talking or not talking about cancer is your choice, and you're entitled to make it.

The other choice available is to take the other door out of the cancer room. Lance Armstrong, one of the best known cancer survivors of us all, talks about that other door as being 'the obligation of the cured'. He means, I think, that those of us who have benefitted from the medical knowledge and expertise gleaned from all of the people who went before us – those who danced with cancer and survived, and those who didn't – should, in our turn, be making a contribution to help the next wave of people being diagnosed with cancer, until the happy day when there is no one being diagnosed with cancer anymore. (Or if they are, they get sent home with a little pack of pills that have no side-effects whatsoever, and they shake their heads and wonder at the days when cancer was any kind of a big deal, before going back to their lives.) I think he's right. But I think that other door is not just about obligation. It's about acknowledgement.

Most of the people I have spoken to about cancer over the years agree that, while cancer doesn't necessarily change you very much, it can, and does, change your life. And because it changes your life, it's difficult not to talk about it. As soon as someone asks, 'Why did you move to Northumberland?' or 'What do you write about?' I'm straight into a conversation about cancer, and those questions tend to come pretty early on in any new acquaintance.

Obviously I have made the choice to be very public about my dance with cancer, so I'm a slightly different case. But I do think that, for many people, talking about cancer is something that both helps them and helps other people. Just think back to the early stages of your dance with cancer. How lovely would it have been to have been introduced to someone who mentioned, in passing, that they had had a cancer and, although they would never have chosen the diagnosis, without it they wouldn't have found the career that they loved/finally got out of their terrible marriage/joined the circus, and they are now happier than they have ever been? Pretty lovely. One of the great things about thriving after cancer is that you get to be that person. Even if you haven't joined the circus.

BAH! THINKING 🐉
Deciding how to help

If you decide that your obligation is to do more than acknowledge that you have had a cancer, and you want to do something, then here are some things to consider before you start. You're likely to spend a lot of time working with your chosen organization, charity or project, so making the right choice at the beginning is important.

*   *What do you want to do?*

    Do you want to raise money? Do you want to work with people face-to-face? Are you thinking more about a behind-the-scenes role? Do you want to do something similar to your day job, or something completely different?

*   *When do you want to do it?*

    Think about how much time you can commit, and when. Are your weekends sacrosanct, or can you think of no better use for a Saturday afternoon than shaking a tin in the high street? Can you give time during normal office hours? If you want to run a marathon, does the event you have in mind allow you enough time to train?

*   *What was most important in getting you through your dance with cancer?*

    You're more likely to do a great job working with something you passionately believe in. So if there was a place or a group of people that helped you more than any other, talk to them first.

- *What skills do you have?*

  Before you approach the place you want to work, putting together a CV of your skills is a really good idea. It makes sense, for them and for you, to put you somewhere well-suited to your skills. I work time and again with organizations that ask me to write and talk about cancer, because it suits my skills and I'm good at it. If I was asked to do a job that involved any level of attention to detail, it would be a disaster.

- *What resources do you have?*

  There are things that you might well take for granted which could be a real boon for a voluntary organization. Maybe you have a home office where you're happy to cover the cost of printing mailing labels, or a greenhouse where you can grow plants to sell, or a dining room big enough to host committee meetings.

- *What are you uncomfortable with?*

  Perhaps when you left hospital after your last treatment you swore you'd never willingly set foot in the place again. Maybe you can't bear the thought of being with people who are dying, or sick children. Or maybe being stuck in the back office would drive you crazy. Think about these things in advance, and communicate them. The happier you are, the longer you'll stay.

- *How long-term do you see your commitment?*

  Some people volunteer for a three-month stint before they return to work full-time; others make a lifelong commitment to an organization and give time regularly over many years. Considering exactly what you think you will want to do can help both you and the charity to find the right role.

- *Is someone else already doing what you want to do?*

  Before you reinvent the wheel, find out whether other charities or organizations are doing a similar thing to whatever it is that you want to do. By getting involved with them, you can make good use of your resources, and theirs.

- *What can you comfortably do?*

  No cancer organization is going to want you to make yourself ill trying to help them. So think carefully before you volunteer for a role that involves standing up for most of the day, or working at a place which means a long commute. Don't let your enthusiasm jeopardize your health.

- *Are you really ready?*

  Wanting to do something isn't the same as being ready to do it. You may feel passionately that you want to work on a helpline or meet and greet at a drop-in centre, but if you are still bursting into tears for no apparent reason once every couple of days, the time might not yet be right. Ask yourself honestly whether you are ready for this. If possible, talk to people who are already doing it. Ask your loved ones what they think. Make a decision with your head, not your heart. After all, if you're not ready today, that doesn't mean you won't be raring to go in a month or two.

In 2010, when I'd been blogging for a couple of years, I realized that things were changing at my 'Bah! to cancer' blog. I blogged most days, and for most of the preceding two years I'd had something medical to talk about. Recovery from surgery, chemotherapy treatment, the way my body reacted to what it was going through, the things I saw in hospital waiting rooms, the frustrations of dealing with medical staff who saw me as just another disease, the frequent and unexpected kindnesses of loved ones and strangers, hair falling out, hair coming back… there was always something. Although I wrote of thoughts and feelings (and the odd bit of knitting, too), the body took 'centre page'.

There came a day, though, when there wasn't really anything new going on. My body was worn and sad, but that was the new norm. The majority of the treatment was behind me. And I wondered whether this was the moment to stop.

I'm glad that I didn't. For one thing, the echoes of cancer treatment hum through the body for a long time, so almost four years into blogging I'm still talking about its effects on my nails and muscles and hormones. But, more than that, Bah! became a blog about survivorship and, later, about thriving. And I found my contribution to the post-cancer party: showing that it's possible to thrive, to find a new life where cancer is a fact but not a defining factor. I became – by accident – a patient advocate, a voice for people who would dance with cancer if they must, but weren't prepared to let that be the be-all and end-all of them. (Or even the end of them.) Every day I had nothing to say about cancer became what 'Bah! to cancer' was all about.

I have yet to have a day when there isn't a post in the blog bit of my brain waving and grinning and saying, 'Pick me!

Pick me!' – which I think is a good sign that I've found my way of fulfilling my obligation. After all, I can always talk about my hair.

BLOG POST, 26 NOVEMBER 2010: THE BEST MEDICINE

Talking to someone about dancing with cancer the other day, I was asked what I think is the most important thing in getting through it. I get asked this a lot and I have, I suppose, a standard answer – keep a sense of perspective, be kind to yourself, ask for and accept help. All of which are true. But I was distracted at the crucial question-answering moment – I may have been wrestling a flip-chart or trying to coax a shy data projector into entering a relationship with my laptop – and so I opened my mouth and something else fell out.

'A sense of humour,' I said. 'That's the best thing that you can take into cancer with you.' The person I was talking to gave me an odd look, and I felt bad that I hadn't given the answer I would have done had I been giving them my full attention. (They were asking because someone they know is dancing with cancer.)

I kept thinking about this exchange, as I tend to when I feel I haven't done something well. (Did I mention that I failed my driving test? Nearly over it. Nearly.) And as I did, I started to wonder whether my response was really that far off.

After all, funny stuff happens, even on the darkest days in life. When my grandmother died, the house was swamped with condolence cards. Two of them were the same. On the day of the funeral, one of my little cousins came in and said excitedly, 'Oooh, look, we've got a swap.' Laughing on – and at – those days is good for you, physically – unless you've got stitches – and mentally.

I got the giggles when a doctor asked me, 'And apart from the cancer, are you in good health?' My Mum and I didn't dare look at each other as a nurse, due to check my dressings a week after surgery, appeared unable to put on a pair of surgical gloves. A doctor writing 'This one' with a felt tip pen on your shoulder, with an arrow drawn down to your breast, before you go in to have a cancer removed? C'mon, that's hilarious. There are a whole load of oncologist jokes quietly doing the rounds of the bald and pale in waiting rooms around the world. (My favourite: Why are coffins nailed shut? To stop oncologists from getting in and giving you one last dose of chemo to be on the safe side.)

I wasn't keeping score, but I'm fairly sure I laughed more than I cried during cancer treatment, and doing it made me feel that life was still good. So maybe my tip-of-the-top-of-the-head-when-I-wasn't-looking advice wasn't so bad after all.

BAH! THINKING 🐉

Getting it out of your system

Take some writing paper – a lot of writing paper – and an envelope.

Find a table in a place where you won't be disturbed, and take a deep breath.

At the top of the first sheet of paper, write 'Dear cancer…'

This is your chance to tell cancer exactly what you think of it.

You might want to have a good long rant. There might be a mixture of thanks and regrets. You might want to tell cancer exactly how you feel – or tell it what's wrong with it. It doesn't matter. This is an exercise in getting all of your feelings out in one go, without too much processing or refinement.

If you don't write letters very often, or if you're not sure where to start, here are some ideas. None of them is compulsory.

Dear cancer…

When you first came into my life…

When I realized what you were…

You made me feel…

The worst thing you did to me was…

Something I really ought to thank you for is…

I'm going to give you a piece of advice…

When you have said every single thing you want to say to cancer, read through your letter. Read it aloud, if you want to. Then put it in the envelope.

What happens next is up to you. You might want to put it in a drawer and forget about it. You might show it to someone else. You might burn it. You might make a note in your diary to read it in six months or a year. Do what feels right for you.

And enjoy the fact that you've had the last word with cancer.

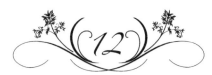

12

Resting place:
It's quiet here

*'I'm not sure cancer changed me as much
as it made me realize who I am and be
truthful to my core. I have more confidence
now in myself and [am] more forgiving and
nurturing to myself than I was.'*
Natalie, diagnosed with breast cancer in 1993

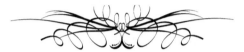

One of the questions I am most often asked these days is: has cancer changed you? And the answer – as with so many cancer-answers – isn't a simple one. It's yes… and no.

Yes, I'm more assertive. I trust my instincts. I've become fearless: one of the worst things that could happen has happened, something I never would have imagined I could cope with, and yet I have lived to tell the tale. (As you know from reading this far, I'm using the word 'fearless' under advisement. You still couldn't pay me enough to get me on a roller coaster that goes upside down, bungee jump, or have any area larger than my eyebrows waxed.) I don't worry, or catastrophize, in the way that I used to, and I use my time carefully because it's cherished and I know there's a limit to how much of it I've got. I laugh more and I treasure the friends that I have – my circle is smaller these days, everyone in it one of the precious people who watched and applauded as I danced, and glared beadily at cancer on my behalf.

And no. Ask anyone who knows me whether my dance with cancer has made me different, and they'll screw up their face and say, 'No, not really, I don't think it has.'

I think what happens is this. I think cancer tempers you, in the way that gold or steel is tempered, the heat of the fire burning all of the impurities away. Cancer, I think, has made me more myself. Not a better person, or a nicer one, necessarily, just someone who had limited resources for a while, which meant that what she is now is the essence of her, and what has gone was never really needed anyway, like those assorted necklaces and earrings, unworn for decades, nestled and knotted at the bottom of your jewellery box.

BAH! THINKING 🐉

Getting to know you (again)

It's possible – especially if your dance with cancer has prompted you to end relationships, change jobs, move house or make other radical changes to your life – that you feel a little unfamiliar with yourself. If so, try this.

Email everyone you know and trust and ask them which three words they would have used to describe you before cancer – and which three words they would use now. Explain that you aren't on an ego-trip, you're just trying to come to understand how your dance with cancer changed you, and you'd like their help. They can repeat words in both lists if they want to. They don't need to explain or justify. (I'm assuming that these are good people who have good things to say about you, so their responses won't amount to a three-word character assassination.)

While you wait for the responses, write down your own three 'before-words' and 'after-words'. (If this feels too difficult, write down as many before-words and after-words as you can, then look at the lists and asterisk the three that strike you as truest.)

When the responses come in, take your notebook and a double-page spread, and write 'Before' on the left-hand page and 'After' on the right-hand side. Start by writing your three words on their respective pages. Then add the words of the people who love you. One response = one word written down, so if five people say that you were 'funny' before cancer, then write down 'funny' five separate times.

What you will end up with is a sense of the before-cancer you and the thriving-after-cancer you. Look at it. Accept it for what it is: an unscientific, essentially truthful picture of you, painted by the people you love.

One of the things I really enjoy about my thriving life – and it might have happened without cancer, as a product of age and wisdom, but I doubt it somehow – is that I have a real sense of all the things that life is too short for. And I mean too short even if I live to be 117. Here are some of the things I just don't do anymore.

1. Read books that bore me. Authors, you now have 30 pages to make me love your work – 50 if I'm feeling generous or am on a train with no other book and no knitting. (This scenario is unlikely, I grant you.) Before

cancer I used to consider it a point of honour to get to the end of a book, no matter how much I wasn't enjoying it. Now I'm ruthless. And the criterion is enjoyment, not worthiness, and not how much I feel as though I *ought* to read a particular book.

2. Doing things that will knock out most of the next day, unless they really, really matter. No more staying up until 1 a.m. watching the end of a film that grabbed my attention briefly after the news. No drinking wine until 2 a.m. unless the conversation that goes with it is brilliant. (My Auntie Susan and I agree that the most effective way to torture us wouldn't be rat- or fingernail-based: we'd give up any state secret you wanted if you threatened us with not being allowed to go to bed.)

3. Counting calories. I know that oatcakes are better for me than cupcakes most of the time, and that if I want to keep on wearing my 10-year-old evening dress when the occasion demands, I need to eat fewer cupcakes than I do oatcakes. I don't need any more detail than that, thank you very much.

4. Buying clothes for the person I sometimes wish I was, or want to be, rather than the person I am. Put me in something too fussy and I instantly resemble a man unwillingly dressed in his mother's clothes at his stag party. I yearn for frills and flounces, but I don't buy them anymore. Neither do I buy things that are a teeny bit tight (because I might lose weight) or short (because – um – I might shrink) because they are perfect in all other respects. And, while we're on the subject of clothes, I no longer iron anything that isn't super-tailored or super-

creased. (So I just don't buy linen clothes. No matter how otherwise perfect they are.)

5. Fretting. If something is worrying me then I go and get the information that will allow me to either stop fretting because there isn't really a problem, or understand the problem and start to solve it. Obviously there are times when it isn't that simple, and either there's no more information to be had, or no immediate solution. But if I've discovered that, then at least I can relax a little bit, and the fretting seems to fade.

6. Being competitive. I do the best that I can. Doing it better than the next woman isn't relevant.

7. Hoarding. I was never much of a hoarder before, but I'm ruthless now. I think I want life to be simpler. And, without being maudlin about it, I'm much more aware of the fact that I'm going to die sometime, and when I do, some poor grieving souls are going to have to go through everything that was mine and decide what to do with it. I want that process to be as simple as possible. Throwing away a dead person's stuff is horrible and I don't want my family to have to do any more of it than they have to.

8. Wishing I was different. I know I'm not perfect; I know I could improve, and I hope that as I thrive some of the bits of me that catch and snag will continue to be rubbed away. But I no longer wish I was thinner/sportier/ had more attention to detail. Apart from being pointless, it makes me forget to appreciate my curves/excellent sedentary skills, like knitting and writing/ability to see the big picture.

I suppose what I'm saying here is that I've realized that everything in life is a choice, whether it's a choice to do or not to do something. And the things that I choose not to do contribute a lot to my sense of wellbeing.

BAH! THINKING

A visualization for being at peace

Find somewhere quiet and still, and become quiet and still yourself. Take some deep, slow breaths, close your eyes and keep breathing slowly until you feel relaxed.

Find yourself in a beautiful place. It might be a hilltop or a beach or a forest or bobbing in a boat on a lake or sitting in your own garden. It doesn't matter. The important thing is that you are the only person there.

Everything around you is perfect. The air is the right temperature. The view is just as you would wish. As you sit – or stand, or walk – in this perfect place in your mind, you feel as calm and beautiful within as the landscape that surrounds you.

Enjoy this feeling of peace. Feel a little bit of it unfurl from your surroundings and furl itself into a part of your body: the pit of your stomach, the crook of your kidney, the space around your heart.

When you are ready, open your eyes.

As you go about your life, remember that little bit of peace that's nuzzled somewhere within you.

BAH! THINKING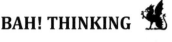
An exercise in gratitude

Take your notebook and find a quiet place and a double-page spread.

On the top of one page, write 'self' and on the other page, write 'others'.

Now think about what you are grateful to yourself for, following your dance with cancer.

Maybe it's things that you've learned, or the way that you've behaved, or the fact that you are taking care of yourself. Maybe you've made some changes that you're glad of. Write them all down.

When you are done, write down what you are grateful to others for. Be specific about the people and the action: 'I am grateful to Alan for never assuming that he knew what I needed.'

When you have your list, think about how you are going to express that gratitude. Do people know how much you appreciate what they did for you? Make phone calls, write cards or plan a reciprocal gesture. Make your gratitude real.

In a way, it's easier to show gratitude to others than it is to show it to yourself, but think about doing that, too. Write yourself a letter. Smile at yourself in a mirror. Think of ways you can be kinder to yourself.

This doesn't need to be a one-off exercise. This could be a weekly or monthly list, or a daily conversation with your partner. Eventually, it could become a habit of mind. Which would be something to be really grateful to yourself for. For me, a big part of being 'at rest' is understanding that cancer is not to blame for everything. That a headache is not a brain tumour. That an argument is not based on your partner not understanding what you have been through. At rest means an acceptance that what has happened, has happened, and life is moving on now. At rest, for me, is not thinking about cancer as soon as I wake up in the morning. At rest is good.

BLOG POST, 30 JUNE 2011 (ABRIDGED): MAYBE IT'S HAPPINESS

The last couple of weeks have been busy. Alan and I spent a weekend with friends celebrating their 40th birthdays in Provence, it was Joy's birthday as soon as we returned, and I've been getting ready for my celebrations ever since. I've been writing, too, and the ribboning of a sentence from my mind to the page never ceases to thrill. On Sunday I travel to Kent to work, then on to London to see my darling godson on his birthday, work some more, visit my delicious goddaughters, and then head home. A quick turnaround then it's off for a birthday weekend with my girlfriends, then working in Germany, then the thrill that is Knit Nation. It never rains but it pours.

Of course, I'm looking forward to all of these things, and I will thoroughly enjoy them – apart from the bit in the airport where I patiently explain to security that a wooden double-pointed knitting needle really isn't a weapon any more dangerous than a pen, and anyway, that half-knitted sock represents eight hours of my life, so I'm hardly likely to risk getting blood on it. But there's something a little different going on in me, too. I've noticed it over the last six months or so. Robert Louis Stevenson summed it up pretty well in *Dr Jekyll and Mr Hyde*:

'Quiet minds cannot be perplexed or frightened but go on in fortune or misfortune at their own private pace, like a clock during a thunderstorm.'

I'm not sure that I'm quite as calm as this quote suggests: but I have realized that there is something, now, within me that is unchanged whether I am writing in my studio, dealing with a crisis or dancing the night away. This is new to me. I have very clear memories, as a child, of going to bed on my birthday and thinking as I lay there about what the next thing to look forward to was. I spent many years waiting for the next thing, not sure what to do when there was nothing, always a little bit empty.

I don't know whether it's a characteristic of being (nearly) 40 or a legacy of my dance with cancer, but I'm not like that anymore. There's a place of equilibrium somewhere in me now, which allows me a kind of stability that is new, and good. Sometimes, when I'm doing something that I love, with people that I love, free of worry, that inside-equilibrium adds itself to the outside joy, and creates something deeper and quieter than I've ever known. It's a feeling that, right now, all is well. And right now is all that matters.

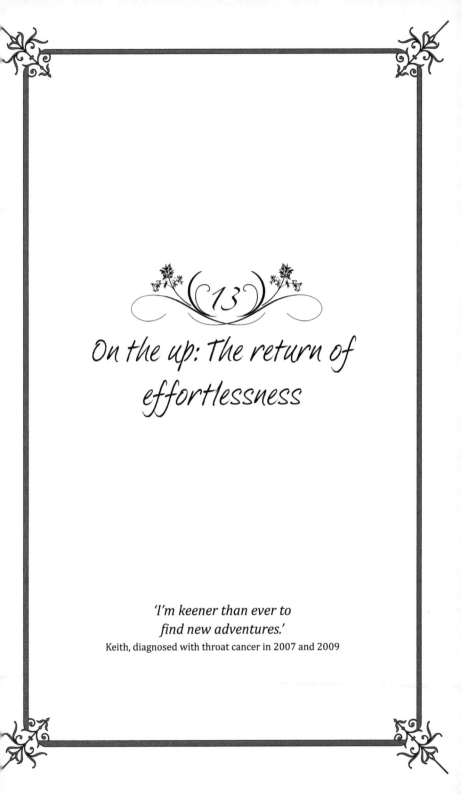

13

On the up: The return of effortlessness

'I'm keener than ever to find new adventures.'
Keith, diagnosed with throat cancer in 2007 and 2009

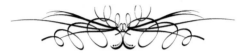

I remember the moment when I realized that thriving was different to surviving. It was one of those times when I met my arch-enemy. No, not Captain Cramp, my other arch-enemy: a flight of stairs.

Those damn things are everywhere. They're mandatory in railway stations, frequently in restaurants – because heaven forbid you should be able to go to the loo on the same level as the one you are eating on – and sprinkled all over everyday life. Shops, pavements, buses, schools, offices, theatres, cinemas, even parks: you name it, it's got steps.

Of course, the majority just trot up and down those steps like they don't matter. You probably don't even notice them, particularly, unless you're carrying something heavy, or pushing a buggy, or wearing a pair of spectacular shoes. (Or all three, in which case, congratulations on your can-do attitude to life. I hope the heavy thing is fabulous, whatever it is.)

When I was having chemotherapy, I was breathless pretty much all of the time. Partly because I gained weight, but mostly because my heart and lungs were struggling with the effects of the drugs. Being breathless is pretty scary. I was checked out by the hospital, but once it was established that there wasn't anything seriously wrong with my heart or lungs ('seriously wrong' in oncology terms being translated as 'not serious enough to stop you from having your next round of chemotherapy'), I was dismissed by my oncologist with her favourite phrase: 'It's just a side-effect.' Oh, that's fine, then.

The thing is, when you're trying to go about your life, and trying not to become a cancer-couch-potato, breathlessness makes things tricky. And steps, for me, became the equivalent of a ring of salt surrounding a snail. I travel a lot for work, and most railway stations give you at least two flights of stairs to get your suitcase up and down before you are allowed back into the world of taxis and lifts again.

I remember – probably about halfway through treatment – standing at the bottom of the steps at a station, looking up and realizing I was crying at just the thought of getting me and my case up there. It wasn't just the effort, it was the thought that I couldn't do this most basic of things that people rushing past me were doing without even thinking about it.

And I remember another time I cried because of a railway station. It wasn't there and then, it was in the hotel afterwards. I walked into the room, lugged my suitcase onto the bed and only then realized that I had taken that case through a busy station full of steps and *not* noticed. That was the moment, I think, I knew I was recovering. I was starting to thrive. Life was getting easier.

BAH! THINKING
Monitoring wellbeing

It's easy to look after our health when we are focused on our health. One of the positives of thriving is that we don't need to be obsessed with our health all of the time... and one of the downsides is that, because we don't need to monitor our health constantly, we can forget to make sure that we are OK.

So, take the notebook, find the quiet place, and make a plan for monitoring your wellbeing.

First decide what you need to measure, or check. It might be weight-gain or -loss, or hair growth. It might be how far you can run. If you've had a cancer in a checkable place, you're probably going to want to add taking a good look at that to your list, too.

Then draw up a chart of what you will measure, and how frequently. Put those things in your diary: first of the month for a breast check, weight on the 7th, and so on. If you are following a fitness regime, aim to keep a record of what you do every time you exercise. Stick to your schedule – and, between times, don't think about it too much. Over time, pay attention to what your records are telling you – the overall picture, not just how your new measurements relate to the last ones – and get help from a professional if you think you need to.

You might also want to add some targets to this approach. That's fine, but if you do, be gentle with yourself. Straight out of cancer is probably not the year for dropping four dress sizes or doing an Iron Man triathlon.

BLOG POST, 1 NOVEMBER 2010 (ABRIDGED): IN CONVERSATION

There was a time when I couldn't get very far in any conversation without talking about cancer. I wanted to explain why I needed to sit down, or was eating Cornish Wafers all the time or was wearing a hat indoors. I caught concerned looks in the direction of my robot arm. I was breathless for no obvious reason, and quite an odd colour. I couldn't commit to doing a lot of things that normal people don't think twice about. Like walking up one flight of stairs, or popping out for a quick coffee, or getting on a bus when my immune system was down.

Then, things changed. I grew some hair, the robot arm vanished, I could eat normally and talk normally again. So I no longer needed to tell people about my dance with cancer. I rejoiced. I saw this as a step forward. I loved to meet and work with new people, and leave at the end of the day thinking, 'All day long and they didn't have a clue!' I imagined myself as a sort of superhero: she looks like any other woman, but secretly she's Cancer Girl!

Now things have changed again. I absolutely don't have to tell anyone that I've had a cancer if I don't want to. But I find that I am mentioning it. Not in a 'Hey everyone, I am surviving cancer' way, just in the way that you would mention any other significant event in your life: when you lived in France for a while, when you had your first child, when you used to work as a chimney sweep. So last week I had a conversation about my old cake-baking business (Cakequeen) and told the person I was talking to that I'd decided to close the business when I was having cancer treatment; and I mentioned it to someone else while explaining the reasons we'd moved house.

I've been concerned that this is a symptom of not being able to let go of my experience, or that cancer has become a part of my identity that I can't function without. But, having thought about it, I think it's the opposite. Cancer is no more or less than any other life experience. And dropping it into the conversation – not as a showstopper but as a quiet fact – is part and parcel of something really important: showing the little bits of the world I move in that cancer is not necessarily The End. It can be just a little part of the journey.

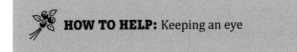 **HOW TO HELP:** Keeping an eye

As the journey to thriving progresses, the role of the supporter becomes trickier. You want to keep supporting, but you need to protect the returning confidence of your loved one. Here are some thoughts about what you can do.

- Rather than suggest that your loved one may not be up to something, suggest a lower-energy alternative, and take responsibility for it yourself. So instead of, 'Will you be able to go for a run in the morning and still manage to go out with your sister in the afternoon?' try, 'I thought we could go swimming together/have a lie-in/go out for brunch in the morning, before your sister comes.'

  Make a mental note of when your loved one seems to struggle. Are there things that they do, or places they go, that always seem to knock them for six? Find a time when your loved one isn't tired and talk to them about it: 'I've noticed that the last couple of times that you did x, you were tired/had a headache/seemed a bit shaky afterwards…' is a good way to start.

- Match your pace to your loved one's. Be sensitive. If they have decided to run a 5k six months from now, offer to train with them, and delay your marathon plans until next year.

- Talk about the best way to support your loved one, but frame your conversation in terms of their wellness, not their illness. Try something like, 'Now that you're so much better I want to make sure I do everything I can to keep you well, so let's talk about how…'

I used to be resentful of the way that wellness after cancer seemed to be a watered-down version of true wellness. I felt hedged around with caveats. Every time I heard someone say things like 'lovely weather for the time of year' or 'a really good job considering that you had no time to prepare,' I was reminded of how I was 'very well, considering', and would get a bit glum.

Then I hit on a new way of thinking about my health and my life.

I imagine that my life now is a walk along a country lane. The lane is pretty and calm and fairly narrow, lined with hedges and plants, muddy and rutted in places. There are no cars; there are no clouds in the Wedgwood sky. The lane is all mine.

Whatever I do moves my position as I walk along the lane. If I am happy, sleeping well, eating well and have managed not to over-commit myself to others or put myself under too much pressure, that translates to a leisurely stroll down the middle of the lane, breath coming quietly, one foot gently and effectively before the other, just in the way that any normal, fit, cancer-free person like me would do it.

If I've slept badly, had a difficult day, have a deadline screaming towards me far too fast, bits of me ache or I drank that extra glass of wine even though I knew it wasn't a good idea, then my place on the lovely country lane of life changes. I get closer to the muddy verges, the spiky briars, the ditch, the hedge. (Have you ever got stuck in a hedge? They take a lot more getting out of than you might think.)

So, when things are getting a bit too much – when I see myself edging closer to the mud and the prickly, stingy bits – I take action that will bring me back in the other direction. I have a bath and an early night. I refuse that extra glass of wine. I take a walk on the beach, or suggest to Alan that we go out for lunch, or go and have a coffee with my mum. I close the computer and call it a day. I take a deep breath and tell myself that I'm allowed to look after myself, and that turning something down is a sign of strength, not a flag of defeat. Because I know that once I'm in the ditch or caught in a bramble in the hedge, it's going to take a lot of effort to get back on the road again.

If I'd thought of life in this way before I danced with cancer – and of course I didn't, because I was much too busy, and thought of my body as a resource to be pushed and stretched, if I thought of it at all – the lane would have been wider. I had more room to manoeuvre before I hit the hedge – although hit the hedge I did, with alarming frequency, sobbing into Alan's shoulder, bewailing how tired I was and rejecting any suggestion that I should, y'know, just go to bed. 'It's not that simple,' I would cry when he had the temerity to propose an early night. Actually, it was. It's amazing how long it has taken me to work out that sleep, rather than pushing on through regardless, is the best cure for tiredness.

Although it's tempting to think that this wider lane was a better lane, I don't think it was. (It might have been if I'd appreciated it at the time.)

This narrow country lane is wonderful, because I know that if I look after myself properly, I can meander along it unscathed by nettles and safe from wet feet. Not so long ago the path I was walking was rocky, uphill, narrow and passing precariously between sheer drops on either side. Awareness of my state of health – physical and mental – means that this country lane is plenty wide enough to thrive along.

BAH! THINKING
Quality of life

Part of thriving is understanding that a good life needs nurturing. Almost anything that looks effortlessly wonderful – a garden, a pencil sketch, the hands of a bride – will have had plenty of quiet attention and concentration behind that effortless appearance. So it is with thriving. If we don't pay attention to the quality of our lives, they can easily drift back into mediocrity. (I had a conversation with someone recently during which they said, 'When you were diagnosed, I would start appreciating everything, and be nicer, and I did for a bit, but now I'm back where I started.' I don't think they are alone.)

Much of what you've already come across in this book – gratitude, facing fears, finding peace – will help you to thrive. Here are some more ideas to make sure you keep on making your thriving life even better.

- *I've said it before, but try to make a point of being appreciative. Thank people for small services. Tell someone how glad you are for what they've done. Admire haircuts, send emails to say how much you enjoyed seeing them yesterday. I'm not suggesting that you turn into a cloying angel of thankfulness, dropping rose petals and crooning over the man who delivers the newspaper in the morning. (Well, not unless he is exceptionally handsome.) I'm saying that if you feel appreciative you should say so. I am still amazed by how often I spend time with someone who will then tell my mother/husband how wonderful I'm looking these days. I would love it if that person felt they could say such a kind thing to me directly. I can understand why they don't: not everyone is quite sure how to address the question of looks/health with someone who is moving towards thriving after cancer. By being appreciative yourself, you give others permission to do the same.*

- *Think carefully before you agree to anything. The fast lane to feeling that you are barely surviving is to do too much, scrambling from project to appointment to dinner date and not enjoying any of the things that, taken at a slower pace, would have given you pleasure.*

- *Recognize your own danger signs. They might be anything from an inability to sleep to a desire for out-of-the-ordinary-for-you foods, sharp cravings for company, solitude or terrible TV. When you notice them, take action to protect your quality of life.*

- *Before you do anything, get into the habit of asking yourself: 'How is this adding to my quality of life?'*

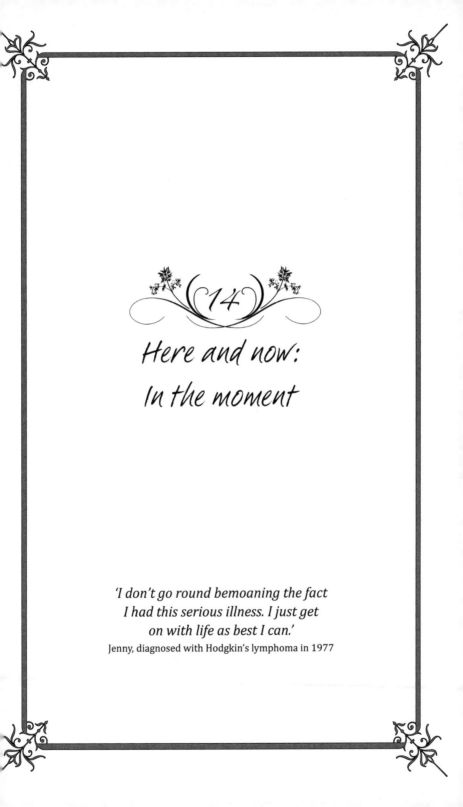

14

Here and now:
In the moment

*'I don't go round bemoaning the fact
I had this serious illness. I just get
on with life as best I can.'*
Jenny, diagnosed with Hodgkin's lymphoma in 1977

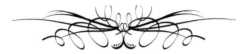

I had a slightly unusual side-effect when I was having treatment for cancer. I ached. But 'ached' is not really a good enough word for it. I felt as though every bone in my body was being, individually and simultaneously, crushed. I felt as though I was being held at precisely the point before the pressure would shatter my bones into a thousand shards – and that the shattering would be a relief.

OK, so it probably wasn't that bad. But it felt that bad. It felt that bad for lots of reasons: I was tired, I was sad, I was fed up of cancer and cancer treatment. I hadn't wanted to have chemotherapy in the first place – I know, there isn't exactly a queue, but because it was more precautionary than potentially life-saving, I really wasn't well-disposed towards it. My digestive system wasn't functioning properly so I didn't have everything I needed to be able to cope with the physical trauma. My oncologist was unsympathetic-bordering-on-rude, and my husband was having to persuade and cajole the hospital into giving me the stronger pain medication that I so clearly needed.

All of these factors added up to the Worst Weekend Ever. And I got through it with a simple strategy. At the end of Saturday, I got into bed and I said to Alan, 'That's a day I never have to have again.' The next morning, after a terrible night, I said, 'At least that night has gone.'

As the day progressed and the pain kept up, I watched the clock. 'There goes another hour.' I lay on the sofa and watched TV programmes in 40-minute episodes. At the end of each one, I said to myself, 'That's the end of another chunk of this day.'

When Alan came back from the hospital with some serious painkillers, it was 9:27 p.m. according to the clock on the video recorder. I know because, since he'd left at 8:34 p.m., all I'd done was watch those shiny red numbers clamber up to the hour and then slide down and start again. And with every minute, I thought to myself, 'There's a minute that I never have to have again.'

This sounds utterly wretched and pretty self-indulgent. I don't think it was either, really. I'd tried and given up on TV and reading and knitting, and I couldn't really call anyone because as soon as someone asked, 'How are you?' I'd sob and sob and it didn't seem fair on either of us. What relieved the wretchedness, in part, was that every time I watched a number click over I was whizzed back ten years or so. Ned, always an early riser, would climb into bed with me back then, and I'd cuddle him in in the hope that we could both get a little bit more sleep. He'd watch the clock on the bedside table and show off his new-found reading skills: 'Mummy, it's – five – two dots – two two.' I'd mumble something and drift off. Then his little body would jump with excitement in my arms: 'Mummy, it's – five – two dots – two *three*.' I'd usually last until about five – two dots – four five before I'd give up, get up and put the *Thomas the Tank Engine* video on.

What I learned from the whole miserable weekend – apart from the fact that codeine really rocks – is that you only have to deal with the moment. The immediate is all, really, that you have. I know that Buddhists have known this forever; I know it's not new knowledge. But it was new to me because it had such a powerful effect, and ever since then I have tried to get better at taking notice of what is here, now, because that's all I really have. That's all any of us really have.

BAH! THINKING

Everyday awareness

Find a space in your day when you can be quiet for a few minutes.

Sit still and quiet.

Observe.

What do you see?

What do you hear?

What do you smell?

Notice one thing, and then notice the next.

Try not to comment, or extrapolate. This isn't about, 'I smell the lilies in the hall, which reminds me I must organize flowers for Granny's birthday.' It's about: 'I smell the lilies. I hear the traffic. There's an ambulance. I see the cat stirring. I feel a draught from the bathroom window. I hear a bird. It might be a crow. I feel how stiff my ankle is...' and so on.

If you practise being in the moment every day, just for a moment or two, then it will soon become a habit of mind, and the more you do it with the everyday, the easier it becomes to do it with the more stressful things in life.

BLOG POST, 28 MARCH 2010: JUST THIS

On Friday I was working in Cumbria, a beautiful (if wet) part of England, and it was a good day. (I was greeted by one delegate with the words, 'Ah, you're the Blue Hat Ninja we've heard so much about.' Have I mentioned that I love my job?)

I was on a train home at 6 p.m. and back in London at 9:30 p.m., absolutely shattered, so I bundled myself into a cab and watched Friday night London wend by. The sky was clear, the roads were clear, the river gleamed, and I sat back and let the pavements pass, grateful for a taxi driver who was happy listening to the radio. (I'm always up for a chat with a cabbie, but when I've been training all day and travelling all evening I'm unlikely to hit any conversational highs.)

I wasn't taking much notice of where I was going, but the streets started to look familiar, and before I knew it I was sailing past the Royal Marsden hospital in Fulham, where I had four weeks of radiotherapy last year. I remembered the walk from the Tube station, the steps down to the radiotherapy department, the sunburned nipple, the daily undressing and dressing for a 90-second blast of cancer-death-ray.

I thought about how long ago those days now seem, although it's not even a year since radiotherapy began. I thought about how well I thought I was then, and how much better I am now, and how much better I intend that my health will be.

I sat in the back of the black cab that was bringing me home, and I felt utterly, utterly at peace with how life was in that moment. Cancer, radiotherapy, Herceptin, all of them fell away and it was just me and my journey, the dark streets, the lights, the radio rattling on, the family I was going home to, and a moment of completeness and happiness and peace.

I was going to extrapolate this moment: I was going to write about how I might not have noticed/realized/ cared pre-cancer, or how important it is to remember that 'this too will pass.' But you can extrapolate that yourself, if you'd like to. Because that one little moment was perfect, just the way it was.

HOW TO HELP: A walk in the moment

If you and your loved one are both reading this book, then suggest the two of you take a walk. It doesn't matter whether it's a 15-mile country hike with a stop off for a pint of cider and a ploughman's lunch, or a stroll down your busy city street to buy a pint of milk. This is about what you do *while* you are walking.

Notice what's around you.

Tell each other what you can see, taste, smell, hear. 'The clouds are moving quickly.' 'Your eyes look extra green in this light.' 'I hear an ice-cream van.'

Don't discuss any of these things. Just keep observing and telling each other what's there.

'I think that's ragwort.' 'I can smell bacon.'

It will feel odd to begin with. And then it will get comfortable, and relaxing, as you settle into your surroundings.

This is a lovely thing to do when life is feeling a bit much. You can do it when you're walking, or on a train, or sitting in a café. It will put you, together, in the moment. Which is a good place to be.

Being in the moment is not the same as being reckless, or uncaring, or irresponsible. It's not an excuse for not doing your tax return, or overdoing the whisky for the third night in a row because 'in the moment' it feels like a good idea. (I'm sure I'm not the only person with a rattle of skeletons in a cupboard marked 'Seemed like a good idea at the time'.) Neither is it about ignoring problems or adopting an 'all will be well' approach while applying for that eleventh credit card. The trick of being in the moment is the understanding that, if all is well right now, if your breath flows easily and the light is good enough to read by and your book is absorbing and your chair is comfortable, then this moment deserves to be enjoyed for itself. Worrying about whether you will get the job you've applied for, or what your mother thinks of your partner can't, in this moment, be helpful.

In other words, if everything is good right now, then everything is good, full stop. Enjoy it.

BAH! THINKING 🐉
Meditation

There are thousands of books – and thousands of experts – on meditation. I'm not one of them.

But this is what I do.

Every day, somewhere, somehow, I find five minutes when I can be still and do nothing.

Sometimes it's cross-legged on the bed in the manner of a Serious Meditating Person. More often it's sitting in my studio, taking some time between writing and spinning, or when I get back into the car after a walk on the beach.

I sit, and I breathe, and I close my eyes. I'd like to say that I think of nothing, but it's probably more true to say that I let my thoughts wend past without engaging with them. I think about my breathing and how it's getting slower and deeper. I follow my breath as my lungs stretch and shrink around it.

And when I open my eyes again – sometimes to find only three minutes have passed, sometimes 15 – I feel better than I did when I closed them. Refreshed. Calm. Silent in my heart. Which is not a bad use of that time, I think.

Very occasionally, I feel something else. 'Peace' seems too trite a word for it. It's a sort of dissolving away of the self: a true sense of being, and at the same time, utter nothingness. And of course, as soon as that happens I get all excited and consciousness crashes in like the seventh wave, and that feeling has gone. But that doesn't matter, somehow.

Please, try meditation for yourself. I think you might like it.

🌱 🌱 🌱

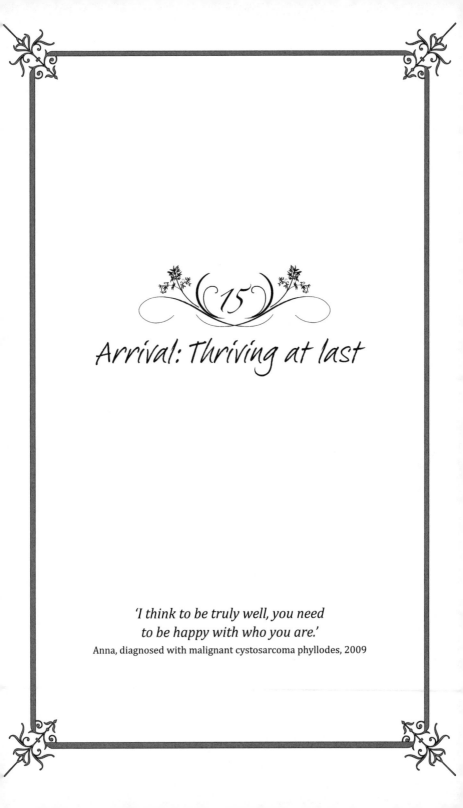

15

Arrival: Thriving at last

*'I think to be truly well, you need
to be happy with who you are.'*
Anna, diagnosed with malignant cystosarcoma phyllodes, 2009

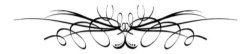

Talking to someone about writing this book, I explained how it was about the journey from being a survivor of cancer to being someone who is thriving after it. 'But does that ever stop?' they asked, and of course they were right, in the sense that, however well we think we are, we never know how much better we are going to become. Ten months after I was diagnosed with cancer, we threw a 'Bah! to cancer' party and I felt fantastic. I felt well, and happy, and Done With Cancer. When I look back now, almost two years later, I can see that I've come a long way since then. I've lost weight. I've grown hair. I've relaxed into thriving, rather than feeling, and giving off, a frenetic air of 'Look! Look at me! See how well I'm doing! I'm really well, honestly I am!'

But I'm glad we had the party, and I felt well then, even if I feel better now. One of my favourite arguments, as a trainer, with delegates who arrive and point out that they actually don't *need* to do this training because they can already do whatever it is really well, is simple: 'You don't have to be bad to get better.' Once we are thriving, there's no reason on this good earth why we shouldn't thrive some more.

BAH! THINKING
A gift

When you know in your heart that you are thriving, take yourself shopping. Go on your own and choose, carefully, something that you can imagine keeping forever. It might be a necklace or a vase, a picture or an ornament. It doesn't matter what it is, or how expensive (or not) it is, so long as it will last and you are sure that you will love it for as long as it does.

When you bring your object home, take it somewhere quiet and hold it in your hands. As you hold it, think about how far you've come. Think about how well you are. Think about what it means to be thriving and how good life is. Count your blessings into the object you are holding. When it's full, put it somewhere you will see it often. Every time you pass it, wear it or see it, think to yourself, 'I am thriving.' And smile.

When I was in the thick of cancer treatment, my mind conjured a dragon. At first it seemed that she came into being in my mind because I needed her. I liked that thought: the brain delivering what the soul needs. But when I started to write and talk about the dragon, I discovered she wasn't just mine. She had other minds and souls to nest in. I had emails telling me that she got Emily off the motorway, popped over to see Els in the Netherlands, showed Rebecca the colour of her fingernails. And that made me wonder how long she'd been around. I liked the idea that, somewhere else, years ago, in the days when the cells in my right breast were living and dying in exactly the way they were meant to do, the dragon was somewhere else, getting someone else through their darkest days.

This dragon, it seems to me now, is like a secret passed through generations, a creature scanning the world for people who need her and will be able to see her. She keeps on looking for people to help: she keeps on doing just the right thing, whether it's a back-flip in a clear sky or a snarl at a nurse who can't find a vein. She was never really my dragon, but I'm really grateful that she found me on her journey through the ages. And that's why, when I think of the journey to a place called thriving, there's a dragon turning somersaults in the sky far, far overhead.

BAH! THINKING

Know that you are thriving

Every night, before you turn out the light, deliberately think of three things you have done that mean you are thriving. They don't need to be big things: to you, thriving might mean staying up beyond 11 p.m., or taking a long walk, or not having cancer cross your mind the whole day through. Say to yourself, in your mind or your heart or out loud, 'I know I am thriving because today I...'

Sleep well.

BLOG POST, 27 JULY 2011 (ABRIDGED): ON BEING POSITIVE

I don't think I'm positive all the time. I think I'm ratty and moody and perfectly capable of being a bit down. If I was positive all the time, I'm fairly sure I'd spend a lot of time devising booby traps for myself to see just how long I could keep it up for. ('I've just had my eye poked out! Hooray! I've always thought I'd look good in an eye patch!')

I'm not a fan of the 'positive thinking' label. Too often it's used as another way of not taking responsibility – because it only works if it's matched by actions. I don't consider that I think positively. I think deliberately, and act positively. It's different. If I have a headache, I don't walk around saying, 'I don't have a headache, no, no, no I don't.' I take a paracetamol, have a drink of water and go and lie down until I feel better. And Bah! to cancer, to me, is that same approach writ large.

I was accused recently – and I mean accused – of putting pressure on people with cancer by setting them a model for being positive when they might not want to be. I can understand that accusation: I can remember how uncomfortable I felt when, after diagnosis, so many well-meaning people told me that I must fight and battle and win. The language, the metaphor, didn't fit. So I can see that, for people who find the idea of 'positive thinking' difficult or meaningless, being exhorted to 'be positive' is not an easy or useful thing.

And then there's the hideous corollary: if you die from cancer, does that mean you weren't positive enough? If you'd smiled more, would you still be alive? No. No. NO.

I think a positive approach to cancer, and to surviving cancer, and to thriving after cancer, is more subtle, and more practical, and more robust than this linear idea that never being miserable = always being well.

I think it's about... well, it's about smiling when you can, changing what's uncomfortable, asking for help when you need it.

It's about asking a lot of questions, and being kind to yourself, and listening to people who know their stuff.

It's about trusting your instinct.

It's about knowing that life – your life – is precious, and treasuring it, and enjoying it.

It's about waking up happy.

It's about understanding that life changes, but we can trust something in the heart of ourselves to still be us.

It's about thriving, really.

And who can object to thriving?

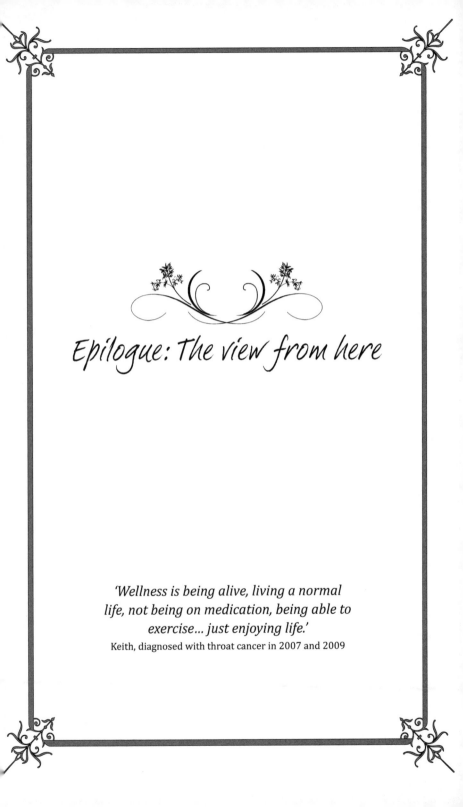

Epilogue: The view from here

'Wellness is being alive, living a normal
life, not being on medication, being able to
exercise... just enjoying life.'
Keith, diagnosed with throat cancer in 2007 and 2009

BLOG POST, 4 JULY 2010 (ABRIDGED): THE BLUE SKY MOVEMENT

I think my dance with cancer has made me more laid-back. I don't get as hooked, or as annoyed, by insignificant stuff anymore. But there's one relatively trivial thing that still bugs the hell out of me. (OK, two things: grocers' apostrophes are still number one.)

Here are some examples from the last week:

On the bus a woman says to her friend, 'We're having a picnic in the park for her birthday, so obviously it's going to rain.'

On the train a woman remarks to her partner, 'If you do get that job, what's the betting that the company goes bust within six months?'

At an event I'm facilitating one delegate says to another, 'I was going to take the afternoon off to watch the football, but I thought, if I do, they are bound to lose.'

I loathe the fact that it's socially acceptable to assume that the world is out to get you. I don't understand why we do this. I hope it's habit rather than genuine belief in some sort of vengeful universal force going round raining on village fetes, delaying trains taking people to interviews, and smashing sparkplugs in wedding cars.

I'd like to hear more of this:

'The whole thing went absolutely perfectly.'

'I'm going on holiday and I think the weather will be lovely.'

'There were lots of things that could have gone wrong, but none of them did.'

We need to get better at recognizing how much of life goes smoothly… and would it really do any harm to expect life to go well? Before I was diagnosed with a cancer my starting point was always, 'What could possibly go wrong?' and I'm glad that it still is. I don't believe that spending 2008 thinking, 'I'm really, really happy and life is going so well… surely disaster is waiting round the corner?' would have prepared me any better for my dance with cancer.

As you will know if you've been hanging out here for a while, I'm a doer, and I've realized I need to do something about this. I've decided against a press campaign (don't have time) or a pressure group (can't be bothered), but I have decided that from now on I will challenge these assumption of ill-luck when I hear them. I might not accost strangers on trains, but I will ask my friends, relations and colleagues why they think it will rain just because they are having a barbecue. Please, feel free to do the same.

I think we'll call this the Blue Sky Movement.

******

Thriving is not the same as being in the place you were before your dance with cancer began. I will never be that woman again: I'll always be bumpier-breasted and scarred, and there's a good chance too that I'll keep on being a little bit tender-mouthed and easily tired.

And that's fine. I don't want to go backwards. Yes, I'd like my old breasts (minus the cancer) and hair colour (minus the grey) back. I'd love some more energy, but I've never really tried to get back to the place that I started from. My dad often says, 'You can only go on from where you are,' and that's what I have striven to do: to move on from being Defeated by Steps and eventually getting to thriving, trotting up a flight of stairs while holding a conversation, and not even noticing that I'm moving up, up, up as I go.

My version of thriving is not going to win an Olympic medal, or a beauty contest, or a modelling contract, or any award that requires my-children-no-longer-recognize-me-because-they-never-see-me effort. That's fine. My version of thriving allows me to function happily within a life that I love, and to do it without needing special consideration or being under peculiar strain.

My version of thriving means time well spent with people well worth it, work that is meaningful to me, and barely giving a thought to cancer.

Except for the occasional pause to say 'Bah!', of course.

Resources

Cancer Books

Anticancer: A New Way of Life, David Serban-Schreiber (Michael Joseph, 2008; revised edn 2011)

The Breast Cancer Book: A Personal Guide to Help You Through It and Beyond, Val Sampson and Debbie Fenlon (Vermillion, 2000)

Love, Medicine and Miracles, Dr Bernie Siegel (Rider, 1999)

Cancer Information Websites

www.cancerhelp.org.uk

www.macmillan.org.uk

About Mindfulness

The Mindful Manifesto: How doing less and noticing more can help us thrive in a stressed-out world, Dr Jonty Heaversedge and Ed Halliwell (Hay House, 2010; revised edn 2012)

One-Minute Mindfulness: How to Live in the Moment, Simon Parke (Hay House, 2011)

Peace Is Every Step: The Path of Mindfulness in Everyday Life, Thich Nhat Hanh (Rider, 1991)

About Meditation

Meditations: Creative Visualisation and Meditation Exercises to Enrich Your Life, Shakti Gawain (New World Library, 2003)

Teach Us to Sit Still: A Sceptic's Search for Health and Healing, Tim Parks (Vintage, 2011)

Teach Yourself to Meditate: Over 20 simple exercises for peace, health and clarity of mind, Eric Harrison (Piatkus, 1994)

About Thinking

59 Seconds: Think a little, change a lot, Prof Richard Wiseman (Pan, 2010)

Teach Yourself to Think, Dr Edward de Bono (Penguin, 2009)

About Depression

Depression: The Way Out of Your Prison, Dorothy Rowe (Routledge, 2003)

Feeling good: The New Mood Therapy, Dr David D Burns (Avon Books, 2000)

About Happiness

Happiness – Essential Mindfulness Practices, Thich Nhat Hanh (Parallax Press, 2009)

Happiness Now! Timeless wisdom for feeling good fast, Robert Holden (Hay House, 1999; revised edn 2011)

Hay House titles of related interest

Cancer (CD), by Louise L. Hay

Eliminating Stress, Finding Inner Peace (book with CD), by Brian L. Weiss

Heal Your Body, by Louise L. Hay

Help Me to Heal, by Bernie S. Siegel

How Your Mind Can Heal Your Body, by David R. Hamilton PhD

The Power of Joy (CD), by Dr Christiane Northrup

You Can Heal Your Life, by Louise L. Hay